HEALING A.D.D.
AT HOME
IN 30 DAYS

Daily Journal and Videos

Daniel G. Amen, MD
Tana K. Amen, BSN, RN

BOOKS BY DR. DANIEL AMEN

The Daniel Plan, with Rick Warren and Mark Hyman (Zondervan 2013)

Unleash the Power of the Female Brain (Harmony 2013)

Use Your Brain to Change Your Age (Crown Archetype, 2012)

The Amen Solution (Crown Archetype, 2011)

Change Your Brain, Change Your Body, Harmony Books, 2010

Magnificent Mind at Any Age, Harmony Books, 2009

The Brain In Love, Harmony Books, 2007

Making a Good Brain Great, Harmony Books, 2005, Amazon Book of the Year

Preventing Alzheimer's, with neurologist William R. Shankle, M.D., Putnam, 2004

Healing Anxiety and Depression, with Lisa Routh, M.D., Putnam, 2003

New Skills for Frazzled Parents, MindWorks Press, 2003

Healing the Hardware of the Soul, Free Press, 2002

Images of Human Behavior: A Brain SPECT Atlas, MindWorks Press, 2003

Healing ADD, Putnam, 2001

How to Get out of Your Own Way, MindWorks Press, 2000

Change Your Brain, Change Your Life, Three Rivers Press, 1999, New York Times Bestseller

ADD in Intimate Relationships, MindWorks Press, 1997

Would You Give 2 Minutes a Day to a Lifetime of Love?, St. Martin's Press, 1996

A Child's Guide to ADD, MindWorks Press, 1996

A Teenagers Guide to ADD, with Antony Amen and Sharon Johnson, MindWorks Press, 1995

Mindcoach: Teaching Kids To Think Positive And Feel Good, MindWorks Press, 1994

The Most Important Thing in Life I Learned from a Penguin, MindWorks Press, 1994

Ten Steps to Building Values Within Children, MindWorks Press, 1994

The Secrets of Successful Students, MindWorks Press, 1994

Healing the Chaos Within, MindWorks Press, 1993

BOOKS BY TANA AMEN, BSN, RN

The Omni Diet, St. Martin's Press 2013

Live Longer with the Brain Doctor's Wife, MindWorks 2012

Eat Healthy with the Brain Doctor's Wife, MindWorks 2011

Get Healthy with the Brain Doctor's Wife, MindWorks 2011

Change Your Brain, Change Your Body Cookbook, MindWorks 2010

IMPORTANT MEDICAL INFORMATION

The information presented in this program is the result of years of clinical research and experience in practice. It is written as a guide to help you understand and overcome ADD. This course, although very practical, is not a substitute for an evaluation and treatment by a competent medical specialist if needed. I strongly advise you to continue any currently prescribed treatment and make no changes in your treatment unless under a doctor's supervision. If you believe you are in need of medical treatment, and I will discuss this topic in the program, I urge you to see a competent medical practitioner as soon as possible.

Table of Contents

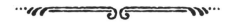

HEALING
A.D.D.
AT HOME
IN 30 DAYS

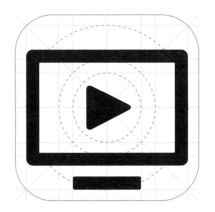

Daily Videos

As a companion to this Daily Journal
you will receive 30 online videos.
For access please visit: **www.healingaddin30days.com**
Please register and type in coupon code: **HADD30JNL**
during the checkout process.

Introduction

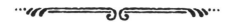

In this program, we are going to give you a step-by-step guide to Healing ADD at Home in 30 Days, based on our extensive experience at the Amen Clinics with tens of thousands of ADD patients over the past 30 years. It's become clear to us that you can make a significant positive difference in understanding and treating ADD in just 30 days, and often even sooner, with the proper information and plan. This program will give you the basic steps of what to do and how to do it.

Given our experience treating people with ADD, we know the importance of getting quick results so that people do not get distracted and venture off to the next project. We have also seen how untreated ADD can devastate a person's life and how helping them get on track quickly provides the biggest chance of success. Obviously the interventions outlined here must be continued beyond 30 days, but if you do what we ask you to do, most people notice a big difference in a short period of time.

Attention Deficit Disorder, ADD, which is also called Attention Deficit Hyperactivity Disorder, is the most controversial diagnosis of our time. The hallmark symptoms are a short attention span, distractibility, disorganization, and often problems with restlessness and impulse control.

Everyone has an opinion about it. It's a myth … it's a fad … it's an excuse for bad behavior. You should take medicine for it … you shouldn't take medicine for it. Yet, when it is left untreated it can devastate a person's life and the lives of those they love.

- ◆ 33% never finish high school, 3 times the national average, so they end up in jobs that do not pay well.
- ◆ According to one study from Harvard 52% of people with untreated ADD abuse drugs or alcohol.

◆ ADD is also associated with a higher incidence of:
- obesity,
- depression
- job failure
- incarceration
- divorce and
- even Alzheimer's disease.

These are not just statistics ... our clinics are filled with people who have struggled every day of their lives at school, in their relationships, and at work. The personal internal terror and shame of being out of control – year . . . after year . . . after year – tears at them and everyone around them. Plus, having ineffectively treated ADD is very expensive as people go to doctor after doctor, trying multiple medications. And the shocking reality is a lot of people don't know if they have ADD. And even if they do know, most are unaware about what causes it and how naturally and easily it can be treated. The good news is that it doesn't have to be this way. We've seen thousands of transformational stories and have solutions that can radically improve you and your loved one's lives.

If you work the program as it is presented here, you have a wonderful chance of seeing significant improvement. The next 30 days can literally change how both your brain and your life work. We are excited to share in your healing and hope at some point to hear your success story. Based on over 30 years of experience helping people heal from ADD/ADHD we understand what works and what doesn't; what leads to lasting change and what only leads you down blind alleys. This program is a comprehensive approach to healing ADD and will teach you the skills that you need to feel better fast.

One treatment does not fit everyone. One of the most important and unique features of this program is learning what type of ADD you have, which will improve your ability to get specific help for your own situation. If you are taking medicine or natural supplements, the program will tell you if they are likely to be the best ones for you. A few weeks are needed to complete the program; solidifying the skills and information you've learned to make lasting changes in your brain.

Through a series of personal and professional experiences, Daniel became interested in brain imaging. In 1991, he ordered my first SPECT scan, which is the study we do in our clinics. Our imaging work opened a whole new world of understanding and help for our patients. We learned that ADD was not a single or simple disorder, that there were 7 different types, and that each type required an individual treatment plan. We also learned through imaging that physical exercise, fish oil, and thinking exercises — not just medications — could change and heal the brain. It was through our clinical work for the past 30 years, brain imaging work, and our personal experiences that we have developed this program for you.

Unique Features

There are many features about this program that make it truly unique.

◆ First, you will learn that ADD is a not a single, simple, or separate disorder. Based on our extensive brain imaging work at the Amen Clinics, Inc. we have discovered that there are 7 different types of ADD. Understanding which type or types you have is critical to getting the right treatment. One treatment does not fit everyone, and in fact, treatments for one type often make the other types worse, sometimes dramatically so. On day one you will take the "Amen Clinics ADD Type Questionnaire" to see what type or types you or a loved one has.

◆ Second, you will learn the mantra "skills, not just pills." Our brain imaging work has shown that there are many non-medicine ways to enhance brain function and conquer ADD. Learning these skills is essential to lifelong healing. Plus, the less medicine you take and the more skills you build means fewer side effects, more self-control, and less overall expense.

◆ Third, you can do the majority of this program in the privacy of your own home. Many of us are too busy or too embarrassed to seek help. I have tried to streamline the process whenever possible.

◆ Fourth, your healing will have a ripple effect on others in your life. One of the reasons I became a psychiatrist is: if what I do works for my patients, it not only affects them, it also affects their children... and their children's children. When you are your best, you influence everyone around you, even the people you will never meet in the future.

You Are Not Alone!

ADD is a major public health problem that is reaching epidemic levels in the United States and worldwide. According to the Center for Disease Control, 20% of boys have been diagnosed with it and 11% of people overall. It has increased 53% in the last decade alone.

You Are Not Weak!

Until recently, many people felt that ADD was the result of a weak will, laziness or a bad character. Recent brain science has clearly revealed that ADD is largely the result of brain dysfunction. Our work at Amen Clinics Inc. has shed light on the diagnosis and treatment of ADD by utilizing high technology brain imaging studies. These studies have helped us see the underlying brain problems associated with ADD and have helped us target more effective treatment methods. We have learned that ADD does not represent separate entities, but rather a spectrum of problems requiring carefully tailored treatment protocols for optimal outcome. This program is about using the exciting discoveries we have made to help people heal ADD.

ADD: A Brain System Approach

Traditionally, mental health professionals diagnose ADD based on your symptoms rather than on underlying brain dysfunction. However, ignoring brain function limits our ability to be successful in combating ADD and other mental health issues. Based on the Amen Clinic's extensive brain imaging work, we have seen that there are at least six major highly interconnected brain circuits that underlie most types of ADD. Problems may arise in individual brain circuits or in a combination of them.

- **The prefrontal cortex** is the brain's supervisor and helps with decision-making, attention span, judgment, and impulse control. When underactive, people tend to have trouble focusing and often exhibit poor judgment. When it is overactive people tend to worry and have trouble letting go of hurts and bad thoughts.

- **The anterior cingulate gyrus, located** in the frontal lobes, helps the brain with cognitive flexibility and shifting attention. When it is overactive people tend to get stuck on negative thoughts or behaviors (seen commonly in both anxiety and depression).

- **The temporal lobes** are involved with mood instability, temper control, and memory. When they fire erratically people may have periods of panic or fear for no reason, they may have dark, evil thoughts, they may be aggressive toward others or toward themselves (suicidal behavior).

- **The deep limbic system** (or emotional brain) sets the feeling tone of the mind. When it is overactive people tend to feel depressed, negative, hopeless, and have appetite and sleep and problems.

- **The basal ganglia** (deep brain structures) set the idling level for the body. When they are too active people feel revved up, anxious and on edge. When they are underactive people feel slowed down and unmotivated.

- **The cerebellum** at the back bottom part of the brain is involved with both motor and thought coordination.

Understanding these brain circuits is critical to proper understanding and diagnosis of ADD. Until recently, we had no way to look at the brain function of individual patients. Through the advent of sophisticated imaging technology, the application of which we have helped pioneer at the Amen Clinics, we can see and evaluate which of these systems work well, work too hard, and/or do not work hard enough. Understanding the role these systems play in the genesis of ADD symptoms has led us to exciting new information in diagnosis and treatment and a new way of classifying these illnesses. Applying this technology has led to more effective treatment. We do not have to rely exclusively on the patient's description of the problem, but rather we can address the underlying physiological issues and improve treatment outcome. The Amen Clinic ADD Type Questionnaire will help you see what system is likely a problem for you or someone you love.

The Current Approach to Help

Unfortunately, many people with ADD remain untreated, especially in females and non-hyperactive males. The embarrassment, shame, and stigma associated with having a "mental problem" often prevents people from seeking help. When people with ADD are brave enough to seek help (typically from a primary care physician), most receive medication as the only intervention. The era of managed care has forced primary care physicians to treat illnesses for which they have less than adequate training. These well-meaning doctors often take a simplistic approach to ADD, assuming that one treatment fits all, which leads to many treatment failures. Usually, "medication only" treatment for ADD is bad treatment. I often find myself saying that *we need skills, not just pills*.

A New Approach

A more sophisticated and comprehensive approach is necessary for treating ADD; one that takes the following into consideration:

◆ ADD is, in part, the result of brain dysfunction
◆ There are specific types of these illnesses
◆ There are a number of effective treatments common to all types (thinking and relaxation skills, enhancing relationships, diet, exercise, multiple vitamins and fish oil)
◆ Specific, targeted treatments (medication and supplements) exist for each type

Typing ADD

At the Amen Clinics we have discovered that ADD is a diverse group of brain problems that require individualized prescriptions. The Amen Clinics have pioneered the use of brain imaging techniques in clinical practice, and we currently have the world's largest brain imaging database for psychiatric indications, numbering over 87,000 scans. We see patients from all around the world. Physicians send us patients from Asia (China, Indonesia, Japan, and Korea), Europe, South America, Russia, India, Africa, and the Middle East. Based upon our research with thousands of patients using brain SPECT imaging (one of medicine's most sophisticated functional brain imaging studies) we have been able to see the major ADD centers in the brain. Our research shows that ADD is real, brain-based, and falls into seven different categories.

1. Classic ADD (ADHD)
2. Inattentive ADD
3. Overfocused ADD
4. Temporal Lobe ADD
5. Limbic ADD
6. Ring of Fire ADD
7. Anxious ADD

To treat all people with ADD as though it was the same illness invites erratic treatment response and failure.

This program will:

◆ Help you see what type of types of ADD you have,

◆ Give you a detailed questionnaire so that you can identify which type best fits you or those you love. The questionnaire was developed from our extensive database to allow you to take advantage of our discoveries, even if you do not have access to the imaging technology in your local communities. And,

◆ Describe a treatment protocol targeted for each type that we have found to be helpful in our clinic.

This program will be a practical guide to healing ADD, based on new brain science. By the end of the 30 days you will have an in-depth knowledge of ADD, the different types and the underlying brain dysfunction associated with each, and tools to overcome them. If further help is needed there will also be a discussion of how to obtain the most effective treatment possible.

Thank you for joining us on this journey. The next 30 days can change your life if you follow the step-by-step instructions laid out for you in this program.

Step 1:
Know If You or a Loved One Has ADD and Which Type or Types May Be Present

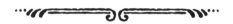

The first step is to discover if you or a loved one really has ADD. ADD is called a developmental disorder because people have it early in life. It is not something that just shows up in middle age. If you have ADD symptoms but never had them as a child, it is likely due to something else, such as depression, chronic stress, hormonal changes, a head injury, or some form of toxic exposure.

There are five longstanding hallmark symptoms of ADD

1. Short attention span, for regular, routine, everyday tasks. People with ADD have a difficult time with boring tasks and need stimulation or excitement in order to stay engaged. Many people with ADD can pay attention just fine for things that are new, novel, interesting, highly stimulating, or frightening.

2. Distractibility. People with ADD tend to notice more in their environment than others, which makes them easily distracted by outside stimuli, such as light, sounds, smells, certain tastes, or even the clothes they were. Their keen sensitivity causes them to get easily off task.

3. Disorganization. Most people with ADD tend to struggle with organization of time and space. They tend to be late and have trouble completing tasks on time. Many things get done at the last moment or even later. They also tend to struggle keeping their spaces tidy, especially their rooms, book bags, filing cabinets, drawers, closets, and paperwork.

4. Procrastination. Tasks and duties get put off until the last moment. Things tend not to get done until there are deadlines or someone else is mad at them for not doing it.

5. Poor internal supervision. Many people with ADD have issues with judgment and impulse control, and struggle not to say or do things without fully thinking it through. They also have a harder time learning from their mistakes.

You need at least three of these symptoms over a long period of time, and these symptoms in some way interfere with your life.

Know Your Type or Types of ADD

Once you know or suspect that you or a loved one has ADD, it is critical to know which type or types you may have. Based on our brain imaging work, ADD is clearly not one thing in the brain. In my book Healing ADD I describe seven different types of ADD. One treatment will never fit everyone. It is also possible to have more than one type.

> You can take the *Amen Clinics ADD Type Test* online at *http://add.amenclinics.com/* to find out which type or types you or a loved one may have.

Summary of the Seven Types of ADD

Type 1. Classic ADD (ADHD) – inattentive, distractible, disorganized, hyperactive, restless, and impulsive.

Type 2. Inattentive ADD – inattentive, easily distracted, disorganized, and often described as space cadets, daydreamers, and couch potatoes. Not hyperactive!

Type 3. Overfocused ADD – inattentive, trouble shifting attention, frequently get stuck in loops of negative thoughts or behaviors, obsessive, excessive worrying, inflexible, frequent oppositional and argumentative behavior. May or may not be hyperactive.

Type 4. Temporal Lobe ADD – inattentive, easily distracted, disorganized, irritable, short fuse, dark thoughts, mood instability, and may struggle with learning disabilities. May or may not be hyperactive.

Type 5. Limbic ADD – inattentive, easily distracted, disorganized, chronic low grade sadness or negativity, "glass half empty syndrome," low energy, tends to be more isolated socially, and frequent feelings of hopelessness and Worthlessness. May or may not be hyperactive.

Type 6. Ring of Fire ADD – inattentive, easily distracted, irritable, overly sensitive, cyclic moodiness, and oppositional. May or may not be hyperactive.

Type 7. Anxious ADD – inattentive, easily distracted, disorganized, anxious, tense, nervous, predicts the worst, gets anxious with timed tests, social anxiety, and often has physical stress symptoms, such as headaches, and gastrointestinal symptoms. May or may not be hyperactive.

> *Knowing your type or types is essential to getting the right help. When considering all of the possible combinations, there are potentially 33 different types. At first this can seem overwhelming, but the interventions are fairly simple as you will see.*

MY ADD TYPE(S)

Place you or your loved ones type or types here: _____

_____

_____

_____

_____

MY ADD TYPE(S) PLAN

Place the recommend treatment plan for your type or combination of types here:_____

_____

_____

_____

_____

_____

_____

_____

_____

_____

_____

_____

Step 2:
Journal Your Success

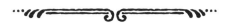

R ight away we want you to start keeping a journal to help keep you on track and measure your progress. One of my favorite sayings at the Amen Clinics is that,

"We cannot change what we do not measure."

In the journal write down where you or your child or teen are each day. On a scale of 1 to 10 (1 is bad, 10 is excellent) rate the areas of focus, organization, impulse control, worry, mood, temper control, memory, anxiety, sleep and whatever else is important to you.

Also, keep track of your food (which you'll see if very important in this program) and your daily brain healthy habits.

Many of our patients find that keeping a daily journal is the ONE exercise that makes the biggest difference in their success.

A journal helps you track your progress. You can flip through your journal and see how much better you are doing—how you have increased your focus, energy, sleep and consumption of healthy foods.

A journal keeps you motivated. Seeing your progress is a tremendous motivator that will keep you going in the right direction.

A journal increases compliance with new habits. Daily

reminders significantly increase the likelihood that you will follow through with your new brain healthy habits. For example, in our journals there is a checklist with reminders to help you remember what you need to do on a daily basis to improve your brain health.

A journal helps you see where you can make improvements. If things start to go in the wrong direction you can review the *Journal*, figure out where you went wrong, and get back on track.

At the end of this program, you will find 30 days of journal pages to track your progress, which will also include knowing your important numbers and motivation.

Step 3:
Get Started on Treatments Common to All Types

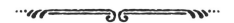

On day 3, get started on the treatments that apply to all of the types.

1. Take a 100% multiple vitamin mineral complex every day. Studies have reported that they help people with learning and help prevent chronic illness.

2. Start taking fish oil. Adults, take about 2,000 – 6,000mg of high quality fish oil a day (1,000 – 2,000mg for children). Research suggests that fish oil higher in the EPA form of omega 3s may be the most helpful. I would look for a fish oil product that has about a 60/40% blend between EPA and DHA. If your type or part of your type includes the Overfocused and/or Ring of Fire Types, it is OK to use a more balanced fish oil blend, about 50/50% EPA/DHA.

3. Eliminate caffeine and nicotine. Both interfere with sleep and several of the treatments recommendations in the program.

4. Start exercising daily for 30-45 minutes. Walking "like you are late" is my favorite basic exercise. In addition, I like weight training and coordination exercises, such as dance or table tennis.

5. Limit television, video games, and device time to no more than 30 minutes a day. This may be hard for kids and teens, but it can make a huge difference.

6. Food is a drug. Most people with ADD do best with a higher protein, lower simple carbohydrate diet. But... not all types. We will address this in more detail soon.

7. In dealing with kids, employees, even spouses – NO YELLING! Many people with ADD have low activity in the front part of their brains, due to lower levels of the neurotransmitters dopamine and adrenaline. As a way to feel more alert they often find themselves as conflict or excitement seeking. They can be masterful at making other people mad or angry at them. Do not lose your temper with them, because it often makes things worse. If they get you to explode their unconscious, low energy frontal cortex turns on and unconsciously they come to crave it. Never let your anger be their medication. They can get addicted to it.there is a checklist with reminders to help you remember what you need to do on a daily basis to improve your brain health.

A journal helps you see where you can make improvements. If things start to go in the wrong direction you can review the Journal, figure out where you went wrong, and get back on track.

At the end of this program, you will find 30 days of journal pages to track your progress, which will also include knowing your important numbers and motivation.

Step 4:
Know Your Important Numbers

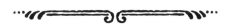

Another very important part of our assessment program is to know your important health numbers. You cannot change what you do not measure. Here is the list of the key numbers you should know about yourself. Put them in the journal at the end of the program.

1. BMI. BMI stands for "Body Mass Index," a measure of your weight compared to your height. A normal BMI is between 18.5 and 25. Overweight is between 25 and 30, while obese is greater than 30. You can find a simple BMI calculator in the journal at the end of the program. Knowing your BMI is important because being overweight or obese has been associated with less brain tissue and lower brain activity, and recently ADD has been associated with obesity, and it is not an association you want to keep. Plus, obesity doubles the risk for Alzheimer's disease and depression. There are probably several mechanisms that create this result, including the fact that fat cells produce inflammatory chemicals and store toxic materials in the body. I want you to know your BMI, because it stops you from lying to yourself about your weight.

2. The number of hours you sleep a night. One of the fastest ways to hurt your brain is to get less than seven or eight hours of sleep at night. People who typically get six hours of sleep or less have lower overall blood flow to the brain, which hurts its function. Researchers from the Walter Reed Army Institute of Research and the University of Pennsylvania found that chronically getting less than eight hours of sleep was associated with cognitive decline. Strive to get 7-8 hours a night. Chronic insomnia triples your risk of death from all causes and is a common problem with people who have ADD.

Sleep apnea is a also a common problem associated with ADD, even in children. If you notice a child, teen or adult snoring and tired during the day it is a good idea for them to be checked by an ENT (Ear, Nose and Throat) specialist to rule out sleep apnea.

3. Blood pressure. To keep your brain healthy, it is critical to know your blood pressure. High blood pressure is associated with lower overall brain function, which means more bad decisions.

Here are the numbers you should know:

- Below 120 over 80: optimal
- 120-139 over 80-89: prehypertension
- 140 (or above) over 90 (or above): hypertension

Check your blood pressure or have your doctor check it on a regular basis. If your blood pressure is high, make sure to take it seriously. Some behaviors that can help lower your blood pressure include losing weight, daily exercise, fish oil supplements, and, if needed, medication.

Get Key Laboratory Tests
Laboratory tests are the next set of important numbers to know. Here are the key lab test numbers you need to know:

- Vitamin D, Zinc and Ferritin
- CBC
- General metabolic panel with fasting blood sugar and lipid panel
- Thyroid panel
- C-Reactive Protein
- Free and total serum testosterone (for adults)

These can be ordered by your health-care professional, or you can order them for yourself at websites, such as www.saveon-labs.com.

4. Vitamin D, Zinc, and Ferritin (blood test). ADD is thought of as a lack of dopamine being released from brain cells to help nerve cell communication. Inadequate amounts of or poor messages from dopamine are felt to lead to the difficulties with inattention, hyperactivity, and impulsiveness. Many of the medications for ADD are thought to slow the body's recycling of dopamine between neurons, and make more dopamine available for use. One step that limits the amount of dopamine that is made by cells is controlled by a protein (called an enzyme) called tyrosine hydroxylase. One thing tyrosine hydroxylase needs to function well is enough iron. Approximately 80% of the global population is iron deficient. Another thing needed to encourage DNA to make the tyrosine hydroxylase protein is vitamin D. In northern climates, vitamin D deficiency is being considered an epidemic. In addition, zinc is needed to help vitamin D bind to DNA and prompt production of the tyrosine hydroxylase protein. Vitamin D deficiency also leads to a lack of absorption of calcium, iron, and zinc.

Testing your ferritin level (the earliest indicator of low iron), vitamin D 25-OH level (the best indicator of vitamin D status), and plasma zinc is an important first step. If you or your child's levels are lower than high average, then they need to be improved (ferritin target of 100ng/ml, vitamin D target of 80ng/ml, and plasma zinc target of 100mcg/dl). Vitamin B6 daily may also be helpful.

5. CBC (Complete Blood Count, blood test). This test checks the health of your blood, including red and white blood cells. People with low blood count can feel anxious and tired, and they can have significant memory problems.

6. General metabolic panel with fasting blood sugar and lipid panel (blood test). This test checks the health of your liver, kidneys, fasting blood sugar, cholesterol and triglycerides. Fasting blood sugar is especially important. Normal is between

70-90mg/dL; prediabetes is between 91-125mg/dL; and diabetes is 126mg/dL or higher. According to a large study from Kaiser Permanente, for every point above 85 patients had an additional 6% increased risk of developing diabetes in the next 10 years (86 = 6% increased risk, 87 = 12% increased risk, 88 = 18% increased risk, etc.). Above 90 there was already vascular damage and at risk for having damage to kidneys and eyes.

Cholesterol and triglycerides are also important. 60% of the solid weight of the brain is fat. High cholesterol is bad for the brain, because it can cause blood vessel damage, but having it too low is also bad, as some cholesterol is essential to make sex hormones and help the brain function properly.

7. Thyroid panel (blood test). Abnormal thyroid hormone levels are a common cause of anxiety, depression, forgetfulness, confusion, and lethargy, and have been associated with ADD. Having low thyroid levels decreases overall brain activity, which can impair your thinking, judgment, and self-control, and make it very hard for you to feel good. Low thyroid functioning can make it nearly impossible to manage weight effectively. To know your thyroid levels, you need to know these figures:

- TSH (thyroid stimulating hormone)
- Free T3
- Free T4
- Thyroid antibodies (thyroid peroxidase and thyroglobulin antibodies)

There is no one perfect way, no one symptom or test result, that will properly diagnose low thyroid function or hypothyroidism. The key is to look at your symptoms and your blood tests, and then decide. Symptoms of low thyroid include fatigue; depression; mental fog; dry skin; hair loss, especially the outer third of your eyebrows; feeling cold when others feel normal, constipation; hoarse voice; and weight gain. Most doctors do not check thyroid antibodies unless the TSH is high. This is a big mistake. Many people have autoimmunity against their thyroid, which makes it function poorly, even while they still have a "normal" TSH. That's why I think measuring the antibodies should also be part of routine screening.

8. C-reactive protein (CRP, blood test). This is a measure of inflammation. Elevated inflammation is associated with a number of diseases and conditions that are associated with mood problems, aging, and cognitive impairment. Fat cells produce chemicals that increase inflammation. A healthy range is between (0.0 – 1.0 mg/dL). This is a very good test for inflammation. It measures the general level of inflammation although it does not tell you what has caused this condition. The most common reason for an elevated C-reactive protein is a poor diet. The second most common is some sort of reaction to food, either a true allergy, a food sensitivity, or an autoimmune reaction such as occurs with gluten. High CRP levels can also indicate hidden infections.

Step 5:
Food Is Your Best Medicine: Get Started on the Amen Clinics 3-Week Elimination Diet

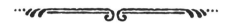

Your brain uses 25% of the calories that you consume and is the most energy-hungry organ in your body. Most people don't know that they can use food to manipulate their minds. Food can help you feel relaxed, happy, and focused... or downright dumb. Here are our 9 Rules for Brain Healthy Eating that can radically improve ADD symptoms, no matter which type.

9 Rules of Brain Healthy Eating

Rule #1. **Think "high-quality calories" and not too many of them if weight is an issue.**
The quality of your food matters, so always opt for high-quality food.

Rule #2. **Drink plenty of water and don't drink your calories.**
Your brain is 80% water. Anything that dehydrates it, such as too much caffeine or alcohol, decreases your thinking and impairs your judgment. Drink about ½ your weight in ounces of water per day.

Rule #3. **Eat high-quality, clean protein throughout the day.**
Protein helps balance your blood sugar, helps you focus, and provides the necessary building blocks for brain health. Start each day with protein to boost your focus and concentration skills!

Make it clean to avoid hormones and toxins. When possible eat hormone free, antibiotic free, free range, grass fed meat.

Rule #4. Eat smart carbohydrates (low glycemic, high fiber).

"Smart" carbohydrates are ones that don't spike your blood sugar (low-glycemic index) and are also high in fiber, such as vegetables and fruits like blueberries and apples. Carbs are not the enemy... but bad carbohydrates are. Sugar is NOT your friend – it increases erratic brain cell firing, is addictive, has been implicated in aggression, and increases inflammation in the body and the brain.

Rule #5. Focus your diet on healthy fats.

Fat is not the enemy, and good fats are essential to your health. The solid weight of your brain is 60% fat (after the water is removed) and 20% cholesterol. Focus your diet on healthy fats, especially those that contain omega-3 fatty acids; from foods like salmon, sardines, avocados, walnuts, flaxseed, chia seed, and dark green leafy vegetables.

Rule #6. Eat from the rainbow.

Put natural foods of many different colors into your diet; include blueberries, pomegranates, yellow squash, and red bell peppers. This will boost the antioxidant levels in your body and help keep your brain young!

Rule #7. Cook with brain-healthy herbs and spices to boost your brain.

Here's a little food for thought...

- ◆ There is good scientific evidence that rosemary, thyme, and sage help boost memory.
- ◆ Cinnamon has been shown to help attention and blood sugar.
- ◆ Garlic and oregano boost blood flow to the brain.
- ◆ In 3 studies, a saffron extract was found to be as effective as antidepressant medication in treating people with major depression!

Rule #8. Make sure your food is as clean as possible.

As much as possible:

♦ Eat organically grown or raised foods, as pesticides used in commercial farming can accumulate in your brain and body, even though the levels in each food may be low.

♦ Additionally, eliminate food additives, preservatives, and artificial dyes and sweeteners.

Rule #9. We believe all people with ADD/ADHD should try an elimination diet for 3 weeks, especially eliminating wheat, other gluten-containing grains or foods, dairy, soy, and corn.

Did you know that gluten can literally make some people crazy? In our experience, ADD-affected and autistic children and adults often do better when they get rid of wheat, dairy, all the processed foods, all forms of sugar and sugar alternatives, food dyes, and additives.

We are coming to understand that subtle but important food sensitivities may result in brain inflammation that contributes to many of the brain issues we see at Amen Clinics, including ADD. These food sensitivities can be delayed in the sense that *adverse reactions may occur up to several days after consuming the foods*.

Conventional medicine has tended to ignore the role and significance that adverse food reactions play in ADD. However, we believe and have seen in our clinic that these foods may create a metabolic disorder that can lead to many "mental" symptoms, including:

• Fatigue	• Depression
• Brain fog	• Bipolar conditions
• Slowed thinking	• ADD
• Irritability	• Learning disabilities
• Agitation	• Autism
• Aggression	• Schizophrenia
• Anxiety	• Dementia

The common food culprits that tend to weaken the immune system include:
- Gluten: *wheat, rye, barley, oats, kamut, spelt*
- Dairy: *milk, cheese, ice cream, butter, yogurt*
- Corn
- Soy
- Citrus
- Sugar
- Grains: *including oats, rice, millet*
- Yeast: *baker's yeast, brewer's yeast, fermented foods*
- Nightshades: *tomato, peppers, potato, eggplant*
- Synthetic flavors, colors, sweeteners, preservatives & additives

What is an Elimination Diet?

An elimination diet is a strategic eating plan designed to remove the foods that commonly trigger adverse food reactions for three weeks, then reintroduce them slowly, one by one, so that you may identify the foods that may be causing problems.

The elimination period allows time for:
- The inflammatory response to calm down inside the body and brain
- The gut to restore integrity and health
- The liver to clear the byproducts of adverse reactions

Elimination diets are wonderful because they are more affordable than blood tests, and they allow the opportunity to better understand your own body.

The Elimination Diet

❶ **For 3 weeks, do not eat any of the foods on the exclude list below**, and only eat the foods on the include list (below). Be sure to *read food labels* and ask how foods are prepared at restaurants so that you can get the most out of your diet.

Foods To Exclude

FOODS TO EXCLUDE FOR AT LEAST 3 WEEKS.	
Sugar	• Sugar
Alcohol	• Alcohol
Soy	• Wheat • Rye • Barley • Oats • Kamut • Spelt
Grains	• Rice • Corn • Millet • Quinoa
Dairy	• Milk • Cheese • Ice Cream • Butter • Yogurt
Yeast	• Baker's Yeast • Brewer's Yeast • Fermented Foods
Citrus	• Oranges • Lemon • Lime • Tangerine • Grapefruit • Pomelo
Nightshades	• Tomato • Peppers • Potato • Eggplant
Synthetics	• Colors • Flavors • Sweeteners • Preservatives • Additives

Foods To Include — Eat These!

LEGUMES/ BEANS: Eat in moderation during the elimination diet.						
Split Pea	Chickpea (Garbanzo Bean)	Black Bean	Kidney Bean	White Bean	Fava Bean	Lentil, Green
Lentil, Red	Lima Bean	Mung Bean Whole	Mung Bean Pasta	Pinto Bean	Hummus	

HIGH-QUALITY PROTEIN: Curbs hunger, helps keep blood sugar stable, prevents energy crashes, boosts concentration, helps with weight loss, and boosts dopamine.						
Poultry	Game Meat	High Omega 3 Fish	White Fish		Egg	Medical Food Protein Powder
Chicken White Meat	Bison	Sardines	Calamari	Scallops	Egg White	Hemp
Chicken Dark Meat	Lamb	Salmon	Clam	Shrimp		Pea
Turkey	Beef	Anchovies	Crab	Striped Bass		
	Buffalo	Herring	Flounder	Tilapia		
	Pork		Haddock	Trout		
	Veal		Arctic Char	Mahi Mahi		
			Lobster	Halibut		
			Mussels	Snapper		
			Oysters			

Foods To Include

FATS: Helps you feel satiated, assist with nutrient absorption, help fend off oxidative damage and degenerative nerve disorders, and aid in brain health, hormone synthesis, and cholesterol reduction.

Seeds	Nuts & Nut Butters	Avocado	Coconut	Oils	Egg	Olive
Pumpkin	Cashew	Whole	Coconut Oil	Extra Virgin Olive Oil	Egg Yolk	Olives Whole
Sunflower	Walnut	Guacamole	Coconut Butter	Macadamia Nut Oil		Olive Tapenade
Flaxseed	Pecan		Coconut Spread	Walnut Oil		
Hempseed	Almond			Grapeseed Oil		
Sesame whole	Macadamia			Coconut Oil		
Sesame Tahini	Pine Nut			Earth Balance Spread		
	Chestnut			Flax Oil		

CARBOHYDRATES: Provides energy and boosts serotonin.

Non Starchy Vegetable:

Asparagus	Bamboo Shoot	Kale	Carrot	Artichoke Hearts	Artichoke	Cabbage
Bell Pepper, Orange	Green Bean	Leeks	Celery	Tomato	Snow Pea	Shallot
Bell Pepper, Red	Collard Green	Lettuce	Cucumber	Zucchini	Spinach	Radish
Bell Pepper, Yellow	Mustard Green	Mushroom	Eggplant whole	Eggplant Puree (Baba Ganoush)	Jalapenos	Brussels Sprouts
Bok Choy	Swiss Chard	Green Onion	Broccoli	Escarole	Parsnip	Green Beans
Arugula	Scallion	Endive	Tomato Sauce			

Fruit: Eat in small amounts

Apples	Cantaloupe	Grapefruit	Lime	Papaya	Pomegranate	Strawberries
Banana	Cherries	Grapes	Mango	Peach	Pinapple	Green Beans
Blueberries	Coconut	Lemon	Orange	Pear	Rasperries	

Starchy Vegetables: Eat in small amounts

Sweet Potato	Spaghetti Squash	Butternut Squash	Acorn Squash	Pea	Beets	Pumpkin

Foods To Include

GLUTEN FREE GRAINS: On occasion and in moderation during the first 3 weeks						
Quinoa						

DAIRY ALTERNATIVES: *Unsweetened* only						
Almond Milk	Hemp Milk	Coconut Milk	Rice Milk	Hazelnut Milk		

HERBS: As desired							
Basil	Mint	Bay Leaves	Red Pepper Flakes	Curry	Sea Salt	Paprika
Chives	Oregano	Black Pepper	Turmeric	Cinnamon	Garlic	Red Chili Powder
Cilantro	Parsley	Himalayan Sea Salt	Dill	Rosemary	Italian Seasoning	Lemon Pepper
Saffron	Thyme	Marjoram	Sage	Nutmeg	Garam Masala	

Sample Menu

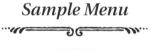

DAY 1

Breakfast: Omelet with Spinach, Peppers, Onions, Avocado

Snack: Handful of Cashews with Blueberries

Lunch: Grilled Salmon or Shrimp Over Vegetable Salad with olive oil and lemon

Snack: Guacamole with baby carrots

Dinner: Grilled Steak with Steamed Broccoli, Olive Oil with 1 small baked steamed broccoli

DAY 2

Breakfast: Quinoa with Berries, Nuts, Almond Milk

Snack: Bring 2 Hardboiled Eggs

Lunch: Grilled Chicken over vegetable salad with olive oil and lemon

Snack: Almond butter or Almonds with apple or celery

Dinner: Grilled Meat (Lamb Chops) with Grilled Asparagus and Zucchini

② **After 3 weeks of eating only the foods on the include list**, decide which foods you would like to reintroduce and create a simple list using a sheet of paper (hang it on the fridge).

a. It's very important to reintroduce foods slowly and one at a time because adverse reactions may be delayed. Symptoms can occur from a few minutes to 72 hours later.

b. If you have an adverse reaction, note the reaction on your chart and eliminate that food for 90 days. This will give your immune system a chance to cool off and your gut a chance to heal.

Common Adverse Food Reactions

- Brain fog
- Difficulty remembering
- Mood issues
- Nasal congestion
- Chest congestion
- Headaches
- Sleep problems
- Joint aches
- Muscle aches
- Pain
- Fatigue
- Skin changes
- Changes in digestion and bowel functioning

③ **After 3 weeks, begin to reintroduce 1 new food *every 3 days*.**

Example:

- Monday: try a small serving of yogurt – if you feel okay, eat it again on Tuesday — if you still feel okay, eat it again on Wednesday.

- Thursday: try another new food, such as cheese (for 3 days).

- Sunday: try another new food, such as milk (for 3 days).

- If you notice adverse reactions – STOP eating that food for 90 days and log how the food made you feel.

After the 90-day period, reintroduce the previously adverse food one more time (only if you wish) and take note of any continued adverse effects. Depending on your immune system, the avoidance of adverse foods may be temporary or permanent. The goal is to see if your symptoms clear up for good!

Protein Increases Dopamine:

ADD is commonly associated low dopamine levels. Dopamine is a feel-good, motivating neurotransmitter that helps to power the prefrontal cortex and is heavily involved in motivation, emotional significance, relevance, focus, and pleasure. Stimulant medications appear to work by dopamine availability in the brain, yet the right diet can actually decrease the amount of medication needed (work with your primary care provider).

- **Dopamine-boosting proteins** include beef, poultry, fish, eggs, seeds (pumpkin and sesame), nuts (almonds and walnuts), cheese, protein powders, and green tea. Additionally, avocados and lima beans can help.

- It makes sense to eat a protein-rich meal earlier in the day to get started, or at dinner if you still need to get work finished in the evening.

Carbohydrates Increase Serotonin:

Simple carbohydrates spike serotonin levels in the brain and also spike blood sugar within the body. Serotonin is a neurotransmitter that helps soothe the brain and is intimately involved in sleep, mood regulation, appetite and social engagement. Serotonin helps decrease our worries and concerns. The problem is that serotonin also can decrease our ability to get things done by encouraging a "don't worry be happy mindset." . . . which can negatively impact productivity at school or work.

- **Breakfast:** The simple carbohydrates found in breakfast cereals, pancakes, waffles, muffins, and bagels spike insulin, which causes low blood sugar levels in a short period of time, leading to brain fog and erratic moods.

- **Snacks:** When kids come home from school, don't give them a cookie or soda (high in simple carbs) and then send them off to begin homework. Doing so will diminish their ability to concentrate and will set the stage for a stressful evening. Give them an apple and some peanut butter and watch them improve.

- **Dinner:** If you want to relax in the evening and go to bed early, decrease the protein and eat more healthy, fiber-rich, complex carbohydrate foods such as vegetables at dinner.

- **Smart Carbs to Boost Serotonin:** Brain-healthy foods that tend to boost serotonin include sweet potatoes, apples, blueberries, carrots, quinoa, and chickpeas (garbanzo beans).

Note: Type 3 Overfocused ADD and Type 6 Ring of Fire ADD are associated with both low serotonin and low dopamine, with common traits that include worrying, moodiness, and emotional rigidity. A higher-protein, higher-healthy-fat, lower-carbohydrate diet (intended to support focus) may cause people with these types to focus even more on the things that bother them. Dietary interventions need to be geared toward naturally increasing both serotonin and dopamine.

Acetylcholine for Learning:

Acetylcholine is the neurotransmitter involved with learning and memory. Liver, eggs, salmon, and shrimp tend to boost these levels.

Heal Your Gut to Boost Your Brain

The gut is often called the "second brain" because it's loaded with nervous tissue and is in direct communication with our big brain. This is why we get butterflies when we get excited, or have loose bowels when upset.

Within the gut is the small intestine, where foods that we eat are further broken down into tiny particles, which are then absorbed by its lining and used to power our bodies and brains. When gut health is compromised by inflammation and allergies, the body is not able to properly absorb nutrients, leading to mal-digestion, mal-absorption, and a halt in neurotransmitter production.

Signs of mal-digestion and mal-absorption are:

- Bloating
- Pain
- Fatigue after meals
- Feeling shaky
- Mood shifts
- Brain fog

In our experience, people with ADD have poor digestive functioning, due to:

- A deficiency in friendly flora, aka "good bugs"
- Intestinal permeability, aka "leaky gut"
- Lections
- Inflammation

Beneficial Flora, aka "Good Bugs"

- The intestines are loaded with microorganisms such as friendly gut bacteria, or "good bugs" that assist with digestion, keep immunity strong, and help us to withstand stress.

- If these friendly bugs are deficient, either from a poor diet that feeds yeast overgrowth (think sugar), or the excessive use of antibiotics (even as far back as childhood) that killed the good bacteria, we are more likely to feel stressed.

- Disorders ranging from ADD to autism in children, and depression to mental fogginess in adults have been connected to intestinal imbalances that cause increased gut permeability.

Intestinal Permeability, aka "Leaky Gut"

- The intestines are a barrier from the outside world to the inside world.

- Substances in grain and a deficiency in good bugs can damage the intestinal walls.

- Leaky gut occurs when damaged intestinal walls allow food, waste, bacteria, viruses, and other toxins to leak out of the intestines and into the bloodstream.

- Leakage can cause inflammation and can trigger allergies and autoimmune reactions in which the body mistakenly attacks its own healthy tissues (celiac disease, Crohn's disease, rheumatoid arthritis, allergies, and more).

- This damage also prevents the intestines from properly absorbing vitamins, minerals, and other nutrients.

Lectins

- Lectins are carbohydrate-binding proteins that can cause changes to the cellular lining of the intestines and contribute to leaky gut, poor absorption of nutrients (including other proteins), and death of intestinal cells.
- The symptoms of lectin sensitivity are similar to gluten sensitivity, and the two are often confused.
- Lectins are found in wheat, rice, oats, millet, rye, corn, quinoa, dairy, legumes (including dry beans and peanuts), soy, and vegetables in the nightshade family – peppers, eggplant, potatoes, and tomatoes.
- Cooking lectin-rich vegetables and grains thoroughly helps to destroy some of them in foods.

Inflammation

- Inflammation is the root source of pain and disease.
- Inflammation caused by gluten, dairy, sugar, and other inflammation-causing foods is associated with the growth of "bad" bacteria, which in turn leads to increased inflammation.
- Where this is inflammation in the gut, there is often inflammation in the brain as well.

Your gut is one of the most important organs for the health of your brain, so it's important to heal the gut by eliminating potential food sensitivities. To test the theory that you are experiencing adverse food reactions, we recommend following an elimination diet.

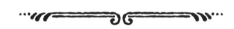

Step 6:

Know Your Motivation: The One Page Miracle

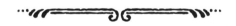

What is your specific motivation to be better? Or your child's motivation? Or your teen's? Write it down and put it where you can see it every day. Be positive or use negative reasons, whatever works for you.

If your motivation involves the loved ones in your life, put their pictures up where you can see them. Write your motivation below and look at it daily.

Positive reasons might include:

"I want to have better focus."

"I want to have improved energy."

"I want to do better in school or at work."

"I want to feel better."

"I want to have better relationships."

"I want to be happier and smarter for the long run."

On the negative side, reasons might include:

"I want to avoid failing at work or school."

"I want to avoid disappointing those who love me."

"I never want to feel like I don't fit in."

"I want to avoid being embarrassed by my behavior."

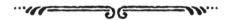

My Motivation

_____

_____

_____

_____

_____

_____

Create Your One-Page Miracle

Tell your brain what you want and then your brain will help you match your behavior to get it! Your brain helps you make happen what it sees. When you focus on negativity, you will feel depressed. If you focus on fear you are likely to feel anxious. If you focus on achieving your goals, you are much more likely to achieve your goals.

Too many people are thrown around by the whims of the day, rather than using their brains to plan their lives and follow through on their goals.

The most powerful yet simple motivation exercise that I have designed is called the ONE PAGE MIRACLE. It will help guide your thoughts, words, and actions. It is called the ONE PAGE MIRACLE because I've seen this exercise quickly focus and change many people's lives.

Directions: On the following form, clearly write out your major goals, in the following areas:

- **Relationships** – spouse, love, parents, siblings, friends, extended family
- **Work or School** – sort and long term school and work goals
- **Money** – short and long term financial goals
- **Self** – physical, emotional and spiritual health

In each section succinctly write out what's important to you in that area; write what you want, not what you don't want. Be positive and use the first person. Write what you want with confidence and the expectation that you will make it happen and include what you are currently doing to make it happen.

Work on these goals over time. After you finish it, look at your One Page Miracle every day, and then before you do anything or say anything I want you to ask yourself, "Is my behavior getting me what I want?"

If you focus on your goals every day, it becomes much easier for you to match your behavior to get what you want. Your life becomes more conscious and you spend energy on goals that are important to you.

The areas of relationships, school, work, finances and self are separated in order to encourage a more balanced approach to life. Burnout occurs when our lives become unbalanced and we overextend.

Let your brain help you design and implement your life. Work toward goals that are important to you. Many other people or corporations are happy to decide what you should do with your life. Use the **ONE PAGE MIRACLE** to help you be the one who has the say.

Your brain receives and creates reality. Give it some direction to help make your life what you want it to be.

MY ONE-PAGE MIRACLE

What Do I Want? What Am I Doing To Make It Happen?

RELATIONSHIPS	
Spouse/ Love:	
Parents:	
Siblings:	
Friends:	

WORK/SCHOOL

FINANCES

SELF	
Physical Health:	
Emotional Health:	
Spiritual Health:	

Step 7:
Understand and Work Toward Healing ADD in the 4 Circles

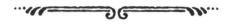

All **great medical care starts with a great evaluation.** At the Amen Clinics we use a "bio-psycho-social-spiritual model" in evaluating and treating our patients. We call these the 4 circles of optimal health and healing. Today, we want you to understand these 4 circles. Here is a brief summary:

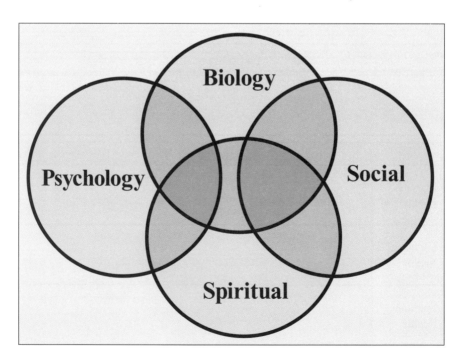

Biology

The first circle of health, illness and healing is the biology or physical aspects of the brain, how it functions moment by moment. In order for the brain to operate at peak efficiency, its machinery (cells, connections, chemicals, energy and blood flow) need to physically work right. The brain is like a supercomputer, having both hardware and software. Think of the term "biology" akin to the hardware of a computer. Within the biology circle are factors such as genetics, overall physical health, nutrition, exercise and environmental issues, such as physical stress, toxins, and sleep. When the brain is healthy all of these factors work together in a positive way to maximize our success. Trouble strikes the brain when any of these factors become disrupted or out of sync. When we do not get enough sleep there is overall lower blood flow to the brain which disrupts thinking, memory, and concentration; when there is an injury it hurts the machinery of the brain and we may struggle with ADD, depression, memory and temper problems; when we eat a high sugar meal our blood sugar often rebounds low and we feel stupid and sluggish.

As an example, here are some of the biological factors associated with ADD. It's important to look at the family history. We know there is often a genetic link to ADD and it often runs in families, especially where there is alcohol abuse. It's also important to evaluate patients from a medical point of view, as there are a number of problems that can be related to ADD. These include thyroid disease, infectious illnesses, brain trauma, and certain forms of toxic exposure.

Healing occurs by bringing these biological factors back into balance, by getting good sleep, protecting ourselves from brain injuries, treating any medical illnesses, avoiding toxins, such as drugs, eating a healthy, balanced diet, getting plenty of exercise, taking fish oil and a multiple vitamin, along with taking targeted supplements or even medication is needed.

Psychology

Psychological factors fall into the second circle of health, illness and recovery. This circle includes how we think and how we talk to ourselves–the running dialogue that goes on in our minds–plus our self-concept, overall upbringing and significant developmental events. Being raised in a reasonably happy home, getting positive messages growing up, liking ourselves and our bodies, height and abilities all contribute to psychological health. When any of these areas struggle we are more likely to struggle with learning and focus.

Going back to our example of ADD: psychological factors that contribute to it include failures at school, work, or in relationships. If ADD is not diagnosed by 9 or 10, self-esteem usually suffers. "Learned Helplessness" is a term that fits many people with ADD, because the harder they try the worse it gets, their brains shut down when they should turn on, and when this happens repeatedly, many just give up. Getting the right help can change the trajectory of the rest of their lives.

Healing our thoughts and hurts from the past are essential to healing ADD.

Social

The social circle of health, illness, and recovery emphasizes the current events in our lives. When we are in good relationships, experience good health, have a job we love and enough money, our brain tends to do much better than when we are stressed in these areas. Stress negatively impacts brain function and dealing with difficult events makes us more vulnerable to illness. ADD is usually made worse by chronic stress such as marital problems, family dysfunction, financial difficulties, school problems, health problems, or work-related struggles. Optimizing your present life; relationships, work, financial situation, school, and health will improve your brain health. Decreasing the daily stresses in your life also improves brain function, so having daily stress management techniques are important to overall brain health.

Spiritual

We all have a spiritual side, where life takes on deeper meaning than just the everyday tasks of living. Having a deep sense of purpose, as well as a connection to a higher power and a connection to past generations and the future of our planet allows us to reach beyond ourselves to say our lives mattered. Many people go through spiritual crises, not knowing why their life has meaning, which sets them up for depression or substance abuse. Morality, connection, values, and a spiritual connection to others and the universe is critical for many people to feel a sense of wholeness and connection.

This is especially true for people who have ADD. When they are in classes, jobs or relationships that are meaningful and important, they tend to do much, much better.

Bio-Psycho-Social-Spiritual Summary

◆ **Bio** — genetic tendencies, nutrition, exercise, neurotransmitter health, blood flow and oxygenation, sleep, overall physical health

◆ **Psycho** — thinking patterns, self-concept, upbringing, and development

◆ **Social** — current life opportunities and stresses, which includes relationships, school, finances, and work

◆ **Spiritual** — deeper life meaning, which includes a sense of purpose and connection with a higher power, past and future

Causes of ADD

◆ **Bio** — genetic vulnerabilities, dietary deficiencies, lack of exercise, neurotransmitter deficiencies, trauma, infections, toxicity, oxygen deprivation, lack of sleep, allergies, dehydration, physical illnesses, such as thyroid disease, diabetes, or heart disease.

◆ **Psycho** — negative thinking patterns, poor self-concept, stressful upbringing and development

◆ **Social** — current life stresses such as school, relationships, finances, work, and legal issues

◆ **Spiritual** — spiritual crises that may include a lack of personal meaning or purpose, a feeling of hopelessness, helplessness or worthlessness

The Amen Clinics Bio-Psycho-Social-Spiritual Approach to Healing ADD

◆ **Bio** — healthy diet, adequate exercise and sleep, avoiding toxic substances, supplements or medications when appropriate (based on brain type), and protecting the brain from injury

◆ **Psycho** — optimizing a person's psychology through correcting negative thinking patterns (ANTs), healing past traumatic wounds, and improving self-concept

◆ **Social** — strengthening a person's ability to deal with stress (stress management techniques) and enhancing social relationships

◆ **Spiritual** — discovering a deeper sense of purpose and connection

Step 8:
Exercise to Make You Smarter

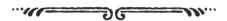

All ADD types benefit from exercise, especially Types 1, 2, 3, and 5. Exercise boosts blood flow to the brain. Exercise also increases serotonin availability in the brain, which has a tendency to calm cingulate hyperactivity. Tryptophan, the amino acid building block for serotonin, is a relatively small molecule. It does not compete well against the larger amino acids to cross the blood brain barrier. With aerobic exercise the large muscles use the bigger amino acids to replenish tissue. This decreases competition for tryptophan, which ultimately leads to increased concentrations of it within the brain.

- **All ADD Types** — get enough intense exercise, such as "walking like you are late" for 30 to 45 minutes, *four to seven* days per week. To get the brain benefit, a stroll won't do.

- **Adults** — also lift weights twice per week to optimize muscle mass and hormone function.

- **Kids** — if you can't find a safe exercise (no brain injuries please… from football, hockey, or soccer headers), take them on long, fast walks. Table tennis is great too!

- **Parents** — try taking your ADD child on a walk (preferably in nature) before beginning homework. You may notice a huge shift in your child's ability to focus!

Step 9:
Change Your Thoughts — Kill the ANTs

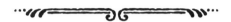

Children, teens, and adults with ADD often develop negative thought patterns, based on the numerous failures they have experienced in their lives. Many people with ADD also use negative thoughts as a form of self-stimulation, but this practice is harmful for their relationships and severely limits one's ability to enjoy live. Learning to question these negative thoughts is necessary, because how we think "moment by moment" has a huge impact on how we feel and behave in the future!

- Negative thoughts often "just happen," so we call them Automatic Negative Thoughts. When we take the first letter from each word, it spells "ANT."

- Whenever ANTs creep into the mind, they must be eliminated or they will steal your happiness! We eliminate them by talking back to them; if we don't, ANTs become the seeds of future failure, frustration, anxiety and depression.

- Some people have trouble talking back to their ANTs because they feel that they are lying to themselves. Initially they believe that all of their thoughts must be true. Don't be fooled – your thoughts can, and will lie to you!

How to Kill the ANTs:

- Whenever an automatic negative thought enters your mind, train yourself to recognize it and write it down and identify the type (see types below).

- Then talk back to the ANT – this takes away the thoughts

power so you can gain control over your moods and feel better.

- Help younger children kill their ANTs by repeating the negative thought back to them and then asking, "Can you be sure that this thought is true?"

ANT Types:

1. "All or nothing" thinking: thoughts that are all good or all bad.

2. "Always" thinking: thinking in words like always, never, no one, everyone, every time, everything.

3. Focusing on the negative: only seeing the bad in a situation.

4. Fortune telling: predicting the worst possible outcome to a situation with little or no evidence for it.

5. Mind reading: believing that you know what another person is thinking even though they haven't told you.

6. Thinking with your feelings: believing negative feelings without ever questioning them.

7. Guilt beatings: thinking in words like should, must, ought, or have to.

8. Labeling: attaching a negative label to yourself or to someone else.

9. Blame: blaming someone else for the problems you have.

ANT	Species of ANT	Kill the ANT
There's nothing to do.	"all or nothing"	There are probably lots of things to do if I think about it for a little while.
No one ever plays with me.	"always" thinking	That's silly. I have played with lots of kids in my life.
The boss doesn't like me.	mind reading	I don't know that. Maybe she's just having a bad day. Bosses are people too.
The whole class will laugh at me.	fortune telling	I dont't know that. Maybe the'll really like my speech.
I'm stupid.	labeling	Sometimes I do things that aren't too smart, but I'm not stupid.
It's my wife's fault	blame	I need to look at my part of the problem and look for ways I can make the situation better.

Step 10:
Sleep Tips

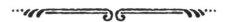

S leep problems are common in people with ADD, yet must be corrected because sleep deprivation is a one-way ticket to decreased brain activity. Getting enough sleep is essential! If you have difficulty waking up or falling asleep, try a few of these helpful hints:

Getting Up in the Morning:

- Go to bed at a reasonable time.
- Set an alarm clock to play the kind of music that gets the ADD person going! Try different kinds to see what works best.
- Keep the alarm clock (or clocks) across the room so that the person has to get out of bed to turn it off. Don't have one that turns off on its own… have one that keeps going.
- Take medicine ½ hour before it's time to get out of bed. Keep it by the bed with a glass of water and set 2 alarms: 1 to take your medicine and the other to get up.

Falling Asleep at Night:

- Don't watch TV or work/play on devices for 1 to 2 hours before bedtime, especially avoid any programs that might be overstimulating.
- Try reading yourself to sleep, but read boring books! Action-packed thrillers or horror stories are likely to keep you awake.
- Try a warm, quiet bath.
- Listen to slow, instrumental music, nature-sound tapes, or guided imagery recordings at bedtime. For some, the sound of a fan works just fine.

Find more of these helpful hints in Chapter 25 of Healing ADD.

Step 11:
Improve Your Daily Decision Making

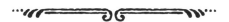

All of the information in this program is designed to help you win the war in your head between the adult, thoughtful part of your brain that knows what you should do, and your pleasure centers that are run by a spoiled and demanding inner child who always wants what he wants now... and not later.

Your pleasure centers are always looking for a good time and want what they want whenever they want it.
Left unchecked, your inner child is often whispering to you like a naughty little friend:

- Do it now

- It's ok ...

- We deserve it ...

- COME ON let's have some fun ...
- YOU'RE so uptight ...
- LIVE a little ....
- We'll be better tomorrow. I promise.

Without adult supervision, your inner child lives only in the moment ... and he or she can ruin your life.

To balance your pleasure centers and tame your inner child, there is an area in the front part of your brain called the prefrontal cortex, which helps you think about what you do before you do it. The prefrontal cortex is called the executive part of the brain because it acts like the boss at work and is involved with judgment, forethought, planning and self-control. It thinks about your future, not just about what you want in the moment.

Instead of thinking about the moment, it is the rational voice in your head that helps you:
- Avoid having a big belly
- Have concern about your bulging medical bills
- Exercise your ability to say NO and mean it

When your prefrontal cortex is strong, it reins in your inner child so that you can have fun, but in a thoughtful and measured way.

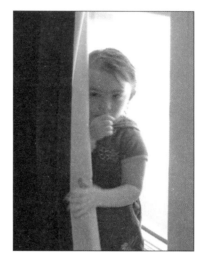

To maintain control of yourself, it's critical to strengthen your prefrontal cortex and be able to send your inner child to time out whenever he or she acts up.

Likewise, it's also critical to watch your internal dialogue and be a good parent to yourself, not one who is abusive or mean.

I have taught parenting classes for many years … and the two words that embody good parenting, even for your inner child, are FIRM and KIND. When you make a mistake, look for ways to learn from them, but in a loving way.

Strengthen Your Brain to Maintain Control
Use the following brain secrets to boost decision making and stay in control.

1. Balance Your Blood Sugar
Research studies say that low blood sugar levels are associated with LOWER overall blood flow to the brain, which means more BAD decisions. To keep your blood sugar stable, eat a nutritious breakfast with some protein and have smaller meals throughout the day. Don't go too long without eating and eat high-quality, lean protein throughout the day. Stay away from refined carbohydrates and sugar… they are NOT your friends!

2. Optimize Your Vitamin D Level

Typically, we get a vitamin D boost from the sun, but because we are wearing more sunscreen and spending more time INSIDE our levels are falling, putting us at greater health risks. Low Vitamin D levels have been associated with obesity, depression, memory problems, diabetes and cancer. It is now estimated that two thirds of Americans are deficient in Vitamin D, the same percentage of people who are overweight. According to one study, when Vita-

min D levels are low, the hormone that helps turn off your appetite doesn't work anymore and people feel hungry all the time, no matter how much they eat. And, it's an EASY FIX. Get your level tested and optimized.

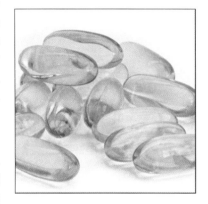

3. Optimize Omega 3s

Optimize your omega 3 fatty acid levels by eating more fish or taking fish oil. Low levels of omega three fatty acids have also been associated with ADD, depression, Alzheimer's disease, and obesity.

Trying to use willpower to make good decisions when your Vitamin D, omega 3 fatty acids, or blood sugar levels are low is nearly impossible.

4. Eliminate Sugar and Artificial Sweeteners and Your Decisions Will Be Better

Eliminate refined sugars, sodas, fruit juices, and artificial sweeteners from your diet, as these can trigger low blood sugar states and more bad decisions.

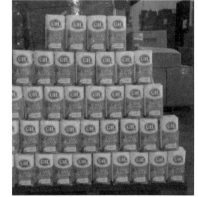

I know this can seem hard because sweets are the language of love for many people.

As children we were loved,

soothed, bribed, celebrated, and rewarded with sugar. My grand-father was a candy maker and sugar used to hang out in every fun place in my brain.

BUT sugar is addictive and it increases inflammation and erratic brain cell firing.

Plus, many doctors believe that sugar the PRIMARY cause of obesity, high blood pressure, heart disease, and diabetes … and all of these illnesses damage your brain!

The average American consumes 150 pounds of sugar a year!!

We need a better way. I don't agree with the people who say everything in moderation.

Crack cocaine or having affairs … in moderation . . . are not good ideas.

5. Manage Your Stress

Anything stressful can trigger hormones that activate the craving centers in your brain and ruin some of your decisions. Chronic stress has been implicated in obesity, addiction, anxiety, depression, Alzheimer's disease, heart disease, and cancer. Adopt a daily stress- management program that includes deep-breathing exercises, meditation, and other relaxation techniques.

6. Determine if Hidden Food Allergies are Triggering Bad Decisions

Did you know that certain foods can decrease blood flow to the brain and diminish your decisions? We want all of our ADD patients to do a 3-week elimination diet.

7. Get Moving

Research shows that physical activity can boost blood flow to the brain.

8. Get Enough Sleep

7-8 hours minimum for adults, 8-9 hours minimum for children.

9. Ask Yourself, "Then what?"

"If I do this, then what happens?" Pause for a moment before speaking, acting, or reacting to ask yourself this important question.

10. Know Your Motivation

Look at your One Page Miracle every day (hang it on the wall where you can see it) and ask yourself if your behavior is likely to get you what you want.

11. Eliminate Anything Toxic

Although alcohol and nicotine may calm you in the moment, they damage cellular activity and worsen ADD symptoms in the long run.

Step 12:
Focus on Gratitude

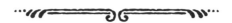

To gain control over your mind, it is important to bring your attention to the things you are grateful for in your life. Modern research reveals that being consistently grateful will have a positive effect on your health.
Your attitude matters!

In a study from UC, Davis, the effect of a grateful outlook on psychological and physical well-being was examined. Participants were randomly assigned to 1 of 3 experimental conditions. They kept weekly or daily journals and were asked to write about hassles, gratitude, or neutral events. They also kept records of their moods, coping behaviors, health behaviors, physical symptoms, and overall life appraisals. The grateful group exhibited heightened well-being across several of the outcome measures.

Focusing on gratitude actually helps your brain work better.

Psychologist Noelle Nelson in her book The Power of Appreciation described a study where she had a brain SPECT scan twice. The first time she was scanned after 30 minutes of meditating on all the things she was thankful for in her life. Then she was scanned several days later after focusing on the major fears in her life. After the "appreciation meditation" her brain looked very healthy. The scan taken after she focused on her fears looked very different. Rather than look healthy, she had significantly decreased activity in two parts of her brain. Her cerebellum, in the back part of the brain completely shut down. The cerebellum, also called the little brain is known to be involved in physical co-ordination, such as walking or playing sports. New research also suggests that the cerebellum is involved in processing speed, like clock speed on a computer – and is involved with thought coordination or how quickly we can integrate new information. When the cerebellum is low in activity people tend to be clumsier and less likely to think their way out of problems. They think and process information slower and get confused easier. When she saw this, Dr. Nelson thought that this was why negative thinking is involved in athletic slumps. If an athlete thinks he will fail, it's likely he will. The other area of the brain that was affected was the temporal lobes, especially the one on the left. The temporal lobes are involved with mood, memory and temper control. Problems in this part of the brain are associated with some forms of depression, but also dark thoughts, violence, and memory problems. In Dr. Nelson's scans, when she practiced gratitude, her temporal lobes looked healthy. When she focused on her fears, her temporal lobes became much less active. Negative thought patterns change the brain in a negative way.

Practicing gratitude literally helps you have a brain to be grateful for.

I want you to do this very helpful exercise in your journal: **write down 3 things you are grateful for every day**. The act of writing down your grateful thoughts helps to bring your attention to them to enhance your brain. Research from University of Pennsylvania psychologist Martin Seligman demonstrated that when people did this exercise they noticed a significant positive difference in their level of happiness in just 3 weeks. Other researchers have also found that people who express gratitude on a regular basis are healthier, more optimistic, make more progress toward their goals, have a greater sense of well-being, and they are more helpful to others.

Step 13:
Have the Right Attitude Toward Setbacks

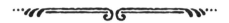

In Healing ADD it is critical to focus on your attitude toward failure. In fact, you cannot fail, because this program is not something you do for 30 days . . . you do it for a lifetime. If you make a mistake, just make a U-turn. Do you have a GPS device on your phone or in your car? When you make a mistake the GPS doesn't call you an idiot, it just says to make the next legal U-turn. If you pay attention to your mistakes, such as you forgot your supplements, didn't exercise, went too long between meals, didn't sleep, or failed to plan, they can be your best teachers.

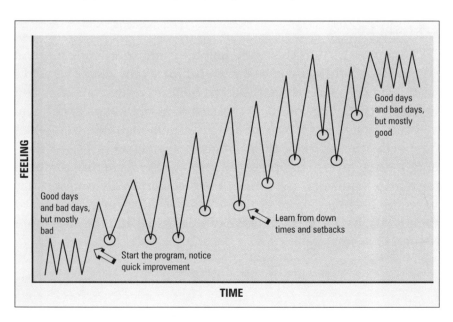

We often draw the diagram below for our patients. When they first come to see us they have good days and bad ones, but generally, they're not doing well. Then, we give them the plan we are giving you and we see significant improvement. We know these techniques work. But no one just gets better. They get better ... have a slip up ... get better ... have a set back. It's in those setbacks that your greatest lessons are learned . . . if you pay attention and learn from your mistakes. Very soon you find yourself in a new place, where you have dramatically improved both your brain and your body.

Learning from failures help you identify your most vulnerable moments. We do not want you to be a victim of your failures, but rather to study them, just like a scientist would do. Be curious. We like the phrase, "turn bad days into good data." Change is a process! If you pay attention, your mistakes can be ever so instructive.

Step 14:
Strategies to Calm Chronic Stress

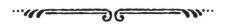

Living with ADD means living with chronic stress, and it can affect everyone around you. You've heard of the trickle-down economic theory; there's also a trickle-down stress theory. When the boss is stressed out, everybody at work is stressed out. When your spouse is stressed out, everybody in the family is stressed out.

Here are 6 ways to help you calm stress to be healthier and happier. Pick 4 or 5 strategies and make them a part of your every day life.

① Meditate or pray on a regular basis. The benefits of prayer and meditation go far beyond stress relief. Studies have shown that it also improves attention and planning, reduces depression and anxiety, decreases sleepiness, and protects the brain from cognitive decline associated with normal aging. In a study from researchers at UCLA, the hippocampus and frontal cortex were found to be significantly larger in people who meditate regularly. Meditation has also been found to aid in weight loss, reduce muscle tension, and tighten the skin.

If the whole concept of meditation seems a little too "out there" for you, take note that you can do it just about anywhere anytime. If you're at work, you can simply close the door to your office, sit in your chair, close your eyes, and pray. At home, you can sit on the edge of your bed after you wake up and spend a couple minutes calming your mind. Try the following Relaxation

Response for a simple introduction to meditation.

The Relaxation Response

One of the simplest ways to meditate and reduce stress is a technique called the Relaxation Response developed by Herbert Benson, M.D. at Harvard Medical School.

Directions:

1. Sit quietly in a comfortable position.
2. Close your eyes.
3. Deeply relax all your muscles, beginning at your feet and progressing up to your face. Keep them relaxed.
4. Breathe through your nose. Become aware of your breathing. As you breathe out, say the word "one" (or some other relaxing word you choose) silently to yourself. For example, breathe in… out, "one", in… out, "one," etc.
5. Continue for 10 to 20 minutes. You may open your eyes to check the time, but do not use an alarm. When you finish, sit quietly for several minutes, at first with your eyes closed and later with your eyes opened. Do not stand up for a few minutes.
6. Do not worry about whether you are successful in achieving a deep level of relaxation. Maintain a passive attitude and permit relaxation to occur at its own pace. When distracting thoughts occur, try to ignore them by not dwelling upon them and return to repeating "one." With practice, the response should come with little effort. Practice the technique once or twice daily, but not within two hours after any meal, since the digestive processes seem to interfere with the elicitation of the Relaxation Response.

2 **Learn to delegate.** People often have jam-packed schedules that leave little or no breathing room. Trying to race from one activity to the next while meeting work, school, and family obligations can become overwhelming. In our modern society, it seems like being busy is a sort of badge of honor. Ask anyone what they have planned for the day, and it's likely they'll respond by telling you incredibly busy they are. "I'm finishing a project for work, hosting a dinner party, making the kids' costumes for the school play, volunteering at church, and going to my book group." Phew! It can make you stressed out just thinking about all that.

News flash! You don't have to accept every invitation, take on every project, or volunteer for every activity that comes your way. Two of the greatest life skills you can learn are the art of delegation and the ability to say no. Too often, we agree to do things without first asking ourselves if the request fits into our own lives. Many people say yes without first processing the request through their prefrontal cortex. When someone asks you to do something, a good first response would be, "Let me think about it." Then you can take the time to process the request to see if it fits with your schedule, desires, and goals. When you have too much on your plate, delegate.

③ Practice diaphragmatic breathing. The simple act of breathing delivers oxygen to your lungs where blood picks it up and takes it to every cell in your body. Breathing also eliminates waste products, such as carbon dioxide, from the body. When there's too much carbon dioxide in your system, it can cause stressful feelings of disorientation and panic. Brain cells are particularly sensitive to oxygen, as they start to die within four minutes when they are deprived of oxygen. Even the slightest changes in oxygen content can alter the way you feel.

Diaphragmatic breathing, in which you direct and control your breathing, has several immediate benefits: It calms the basal ganglia (the area of the brain that controls anxiety), helps your brain run more efficiently, relaxes your muscles, warms your hands, and regulates your heartbeat.

Here's how to do diaphragmatic breathing:

- As you inhale, let your belly expand. This pulls the lungs downward, which increases the amount of air (and oxygen) available to your lungs, body, and brain.

- When you exhale, pull your belly in to push the air out of your lungs. This allows you to expel more air, which in turn, encourages you to inhale more deeply.

Keep breathing in this fashion, and stressful feelings may diminish.

Diaphragmatic Breathing Exercise

Try this simple three-step exercise to make sure you're breathing deeply enough:

1. Lie on your back and place a small book on your belly.

2. When you inhale, make the book go up.

3. When you exhale, make the book go down.

Here's another breathing tip that can soothe stress...

Whenever you feel stressed out:

- Take a deep breath (as deep as you can)
- Hold it for 4 to 5 seconds
- Then slowly blow it out, (take 6 to 8 seconds to exhale completely)

Do this about 10 times – odds are that you will start to feel very relaxed.

4 Listen to soothing music. Music has healing powers that can bring peace to a stressful mind. Of course, it depends on the type of music you listen to. Listening to music that has a calming effect, such as classical music or ambient sounds, has been shown to reduce stress and calm anxiety. Other types of music may be stress-inducing and destructive. It's no coincidence that the majority of teens who end up being sent to residential treatment facilities or group homes listen to more heavy metal music than other teens. Music that is filled with lyrics of hate and despair may encourage those same mind states in developing teens. What your children listen to can hurt them or help them. Teach them to love classical music when they are young.

⑤ Surround yourself with the sweet smell of lavender. Your deep limbic system is the part of your brain that directly processes your sense of smell. It is also the emotional center of your brain, which means that smells can have a big impact on your mood. The scent of lavender has been used since ancient times for its calming, stress-relieving properties. This popular aroma has been the subject of countless research studies, which show that it reduces cortisol levels and promotes relaxation and stress reduction.

One remarkable study that appeared in the journal Early Human Development examined two groups of mothers giving their babies a bath. The first group used lavender bath oil; the second didn't. The first group of moms appeared more relaxed, smiled more, and touched their babies more often during the bath than the second group of moms. Their babies cried less and spent more time in deep sleep following the bath. The first group of moms and their infants also had significantly lower cortisol levels than the second group that didn't use lavender bath oil.

You can find this natural stress reliever in the form of oils, candles, sprays, lotions, sachets, and potpourri. Many other scents, such as geranium, rose, cardamon, sandalwood, and chamomile, are considered to have a calming effect that reduces stress.

⑥ Supplements That Calm Stress — Some supplements may be helpful in soothing stress. Take these under the supervision of your healthcare professional.

B vitamins: B vitamins play an integral role in the functioning of the nervous system and help the brain synthesize neurotransmitters that affect mood and thinking. This makes them especially effective in controlling stress. When you're faced with stressful situations or thoughts, the B vitamins are typically the first to be depleted. If you have a B-vitamin deficiency, your ability to cope with stress and anxiety is lowered.

Make sure you take at least 400 mcg of folate and 500 mcg of B12 a day.

L-Theanine: L-theanine is an amino acid mainly found naturally in the green tea plant. It has been shown to penetrate the brain and produce significant increases in the neurotransmitters serotonin and/or dopamine concentrations. These findings led to recent studies investigating the possibility that L-theanine might induce relaxation and relieve emotional stress. When researchers tested the effects of L-theanine on a small group of volunteers, they found that it resulted in significantly increased production of alpha brain-wave activity, which they viewed as an index of increased relaxation. Pregnant women and nursing mothers should avoid L-theanine supplements.

Servings used are between 50 and 200 mg, as necessary. L-theanine is available in some green tea preparations, where the amino acid constitutes between 1% and 2% of the dry weight of the leaves.

GABA: Gama-aminobutyric acid (GABA) is an amino acid that also functions as a neurotransmitter in the brain. GABA is reported in the herbal literature to work in much the same way as anti-anxiety drugs and anticonvulsants. It helps stabilize nerve cells by decreasing their tendency to fire erratically or excessively. This means it has a calming effect for people who struggle with temper, irritability, and anxiety, whether these symptoms relate to anxiety or to temporal lobe disturbance.

GABA can be taken as a supplement in servings ranging from 250 to 1,500 mg daily for adults and from 125 to 750mg daily for children. For best effect, GABA should be taken in 2 or 3 divided servings.

Healing ADD at Home in 30 Days
Daily Journal

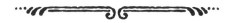

Introduction

Congratulations on taking this important step toward understanding and healing ADD. When your brain is functioning at its best, it will help you get the mind, body and life you have always wanted.

Using this daily journal will help you achieve the best results.

◆ Start by writing your ADD type(s) and plan.

◆ Also, write down your important numbers and One Page Miracle.

◆ Each day rate how you feel in the areas given and note your brain healthy habits and food.

There is also a checklist to help you remember what you need to do on a daily basis.

This list includes:

- Tracking your progress
- Journaling your food
- Writing down 3 things you are grateful for daily
- Physical exercise
- Taking your brain directed supplements
- Kill the ANTs
- Write down any challenges faced during the day

This journal takes just a few minutes a day to complete and will make a powerful difference in your life by helping you incorporate these brain healthy principles into your routine. They will become habits that will give you the strength you need to make the right choices.

Although this is a 30-day journal, remember that Healing ADD is not just a 30-day program. It's about adopting brain healthy habits for the rest of your life! OK, let's get started!

MY ADD TYPE(S)

Place you or your loved ones type or types here:

_____

_____

_____

MY ADD TYPE(S) PLAN

Place the recommend treatment plan for your type or combination of types here: _____

_____

_____

_____

_____

_____

_____

_____

KNOW YOUR IMPORTANT NUMBERS

You cannot change what you do not measure! As you begin your journey to Healing ADD, it is important to take stock of your current physical condition and habits.

1. Body Mass Index (BMI): _____
Find your height in the left column, and then read across that row to find your weight. Your BMI is at the top of that column.

> **Underweight:** Under 19
> **Normal weight:** 19-24.9
> **Overweight:** 25-29.9
> **Obese:** 30 or higher
> **Morbid Obesity:** 40 or higher

BODY MASS INDEX — Body Weight (in pounds)

Height	20	21	22	23	24	25	26	27	28	29	30	35	40
4'10"	96	100	105	110	115	119	124	129	134	138	143	167	191
4'11"	99	104	109	114	119	124	128	133	138	143	148	173	198
5'0"	102	107	112	118	123	128	133	138	143	148	153	179	204
5'1"	106	111	116	122	127	132	137	143	148	153	158	185	211
5'2"	109	115	120	126	131	136	142	147	153	158	164	191	218
5'3"	113	118	124	130	135	141	146	152	18	163	169	197	225
5'4"	116	122	128	134	140	145	151	157	163	169	174	204	232
5'5"	120	126	132	138	144	150	156	162	168	174	180	210	240
5'6"	124	130	136	142	148	155	161	167	173	179	186	216	247
5'7"	127	134	140	146	153	159	166	172	178	185	191	223	255
5'8"	131	138	144	151	158	164	171	177	184	190	197	230	262
5'9"	135	142	149	155	162	169	176	182	189	196	203	236	270
5'10"	139	146	153	160	167	174	181	188	195	202	207	243	278
5'11"	143	150	157	165	172	179	186	193	200	208	215	250	286
6'0"	147	154	162	169	177	184	191	199	206	213	221	258	294
6'1"	151	159	166	174	182	189	197	204	212	219	227	265	302
6'2"	155	163	171	179	186	194	202	210	218	225	233	272	311
6'3"	160	168	176	184	192	200	208	216	224	232	240	279	319
6'4"	164	172	180	189	197	205	213	221	230	238	246	287	328

2. Number of hours you sleep at night: _____

3. Blood pressure. _____

Here are the numbers you should know:

    Below 120 over 80: optimal

    120-139 over 80-89: prehypertension

    140 (or above) over 90 (or above): hypertension

Get Key Laboratory Tests: Ask your doctor to order, or you can order them yourself by going to www.saveonlabs.com.

4. Vitamin D level: _____

    Target is 80mg/dl – Low: < 30mg/dl Optimal: 50-100mg/dl High: Above 100mg/dl

5. Plasma Zinc: _____

    Target is 100mcg/dl – Low: < 70mcg/dl Optimal: 90-150mcg/dl High: Above 240mcg/dl

6. Ferritin: _____

    Target is 100ng/ml – Low: < 12ng/ml Optimal: 50-100ng/ml High: Above 200ng/ml for females and 300ng/ml for males

7. Thyroid: _____

    Thyroid-stimulating hormone (TSH) _____

    Healthy is below 2.5uIU/mL

    Free T3 _____

    Healthy between 230 to 619 pg/dL

    Free T4 _____

    Healthy between 0.7 to 1.9 ng/dL

8. C-reactive protein: _____

    Healthy range: 0.0-1.0 mg/dL

9. HgA1C: _____

    Normal (4.0 – 5.7) Elevated (over 5.7)

10. Fasting blood sugar: _____

    Normal: (70-90 mg/dL), Pre-diabetes: (91-125 mg/dL), Diabetes: (126 mg/dL or >)

11. Cholesterol: Total cholesterol _____

    Normal (135-200 mg/dL, below 160 has been associated with depression)

    • HDL (>= 60 mg/dL) • LDL (<100 mg/dL)

    • Triglycerides (<100 mg/dl)

MY ONE-PAGE MIRACLE

What Do I Want? What Am I Doing To Make It Happen?

RELATIONSHIPS	
Spouse/ Love:	
Parents:	
Siblings:	
Friends:	

WORK/SCHOOL

FINANCES

SELF	
Physical Health:	
Emotional Health:	
Spiritual Health:	

DAY 1

Healing ADD Daily Journal

Date:_____ **Hours Slept Last Night:** _____

Rate	1-10	Notes
Focus		
Organization		
Impulse control		
Worry		
Mood		
Temper control		
Memory		
Anxiety		
Sleep		
Other (list)		

Reminders:
- ❏ Review my One Page Miracle.
- ❏ Take my brain healthy supplements.
- ❏ Focus on brain healthy food.
- ❏ Exercise daily.

3 Things I'm Grateful for Today

1. _____

2. _____

3. _____

ANT Population *(Circle: Low/Moderate/High)*
Write down any negative thoughts and correct:

_____

Write down any challenges:

_____

DAY 1

Healing ADD Daily Journal

Time	Food and Beverages	Calories *if weight loss desired*	Healthy?	How Did I Feel After?
	Breakfast		Yes/ No	
	Snack		Yes/ No	
	Lunch		Yes/ No	
	Snack		Yes/ No	
	Dinner		Yes/ No	
	Other			

Total Calories Allowed		Total Calories Consumed	
		Total Liquid Calories Consumed	

Tip of the day: ADD is real and when left untreated it can have very serious consequences. Also, ADD is not one thing. It is critical to know your type or types of ADD.

Healing ADD Daily Journal

Date: _____ **Hours Slept Last Night:** _____

Rate	1-10	Notes
Focus		
Organization		
Impulse control		
Worry		
Mood		
Temper control		
Memory		
Anxiety		
Sleep		
Other (list)		

Reminders: ❏ Review my One Page Miracle.
 ❏ Take my brain healthy supplements.
 ❏ Focus on brain healthy food.
 ❏ Exercise daily.

3 Things I'm Grateful for Today

1. _____

2. _____

3. _____

ANT Population *(Circle: Low/Moderate/High)*
Write down any negative thoughts and correct:

_____

Write down any challenges:

_____

Healing ADD Daily Journal

Time	Food and Beverages	Calories *if weight loss desired*	Healthy?	How Did I Feel After?
	Breakfast		Yes/ No	
	Snack		Yes/ No	
	Lunch		Yes/ No	
	Snack		Yes/ No	
	Dinner		Yes/ No	
	Other			

Total Calories Allowed		Total Calories Consumed	
		Total Liquid Calories Consumed	

Tip of the day: You cannot change what you do not measure.
Journal your progress to stay on track.

DAY 3 **Healing ADD Daily Journal**

Date: _____ Hours Slept Last Night: _____

Rate	1-10	Notes
Focus		
Organization		
Impulse control		
Worry		
Mood		
Temper control		
Memory		
Anxiety		
Sleep		
Other (list)		

Reminders: ❏ Review my One Page Miracle.
❏ Take my brain healthy supplements.
❏ Focus on brain healthy food.
❏ Exercise daily.

3 Things I'm Grateful for Today

1. _____

2. _____

3. _____

ANT Population *(Circle: Low/Moderate/High)*
Write down any negative thoughts and correct:

_____

Write down any challenges:

_____

Healing ADD Daily Journal

Time	Food and Beverages	Calories *if weight loss desired*	Healthy?	How Did I Feel After?
	Breakfast		Yes/ No	
	Snack		Yes/ No	
	Lunch		Yes/ No	
	Snack		Yes/ No	
	Dinner		Yes/ No	
	Other			

Total Calories Allowed		Total Calories Consumed	
		Total Liquid Calories Consumed	

Tip of the day: Treatments common to all ADD types include a multiple vitamin, high quality fish oil, exercise, eliminating caffeine and nicotine, as well as limiting TV and video games. Plus, no yelling

DAY 4 — Healing ADD Daily Journal

Date:_____ Hours Slept Last Night: _____

Rate	1-10	Notes
Focus		
Organization		
Impulse control		
Worry		
Mood		
Temper control		
Memory		
Anxiety		
Sleep		
Other (list)		

Reminders:
- ❏ Review my One Page Miracle.
- ❏ Take my brain healthy supplements.
- ❏ Focus on brain healthy food.
- ❏ Exercise daily.

3 Things I'm Grateful for Today

1. _____

2. _____

3. _____

ANT Population *(Circle: Low/Moderate/High)*

Write down any negative thoughts and correct:

_____

Write down any challenges:

_____

DAY 4 Healing ADD Daily Journal

Time	Food and Beverages	Calories *if weight loss desired*	Healthy?	How Did I Feel After?
	Breakfast		Yes/ No	
	Snack		Yes/ No	
	Lunch		Yes/ No	
	Snack		Yes/ No	
	Dinner		Yes/ No	
	Other			

Total Calories Allowed		Total Calories Consumed	
		Total Liquid Calories Consumed	

Tip of the day: Know your important numbers.

DAY 5 — Healing ADD Daily Journal

Date:_____ Hours Slept Last Night: _____

Rate	1-10	Notes
Focus		
Organization		
Impulse control		
Worry		
Mood		
Temper control		
Memory		
Anxiety		
Sleep		
Other (list)		

Reminders:
- ❏ Review my One Page Miracle.
- ❏ Take my brain healthy supplements.
- ❏ Focus on brain healthy food.
- ❏ Exercise daily.

3 Things I'm Grateful for Today

1. _____

2. _____

3. _____

ANT Population *(Circle: Low/Moderate/High)*
Write down any negative thoughts and correct:

_____

Write down any challenges:

_____

DAY 5 **Healing ADD Daily Journal**

Time	Food and Beverages	Calories *if weight loss desired*	Healthy?	How Did I Feel After?
	Breakfast		Yes/ No	
	Snack		Yes/ No	
	Lunch		Yes/ No	
	Snack		Yes/ No	
	Dinner		Yes/ No	
	Other			
	~			

Total Calories Allowed		Total Calories Consumed	
		Total Liquid Calories Consumed	

Tip of the day: Your brain uses 25% of the calories you consume. A fast food diet equals a fast food mind.

Healing ADD Daily Journal

Date:_____ Hours Slept Last Night: _____

Rate	1-10	Notes
Focus		
Organization		
Impulse control		
Worry		
Mood		
Temper control		
Memory		
Anxiety		
Sleep		
Other (list)		

Reminders: ❏ Review my One Page Miracle.

❏ Take my brain healthy supplements.

❏ Focus on brain healthy food.

❏ Exercise daily.

3 Things I'm Grateful for Today

1. _____

2. _____

3. _____

ANT Population *(Circle: Low/Moderate/High)*
Write down any negative thoughts and correct:

_____

Write down any challenges:

_____

DAY 6

Healing ADD Daily Journal

Time	Food and Beverages	Calories *if weight loss desired*	Healthy?	How Did I Feel After?
	Breakfast		Yes/ No	
	Snack		Yes/ No	
	Lunch		Yes/ No	
	Snack		Yes/ No	
	Dinner		Yes/ No	
	Other			

Total Calories Allowed		Total Calories Consumed	
		Total Liquid Calories Consumed	

Tip of the day: Eliminate anything that hurts your brain.

DAY 7 **Healing ADD Daily Journal**

Date:_____ Hours Slept Last Night:_____

Rate	1-10	Notes
Focus		
Organization		
Impulse control		
Worry		
Mood		
Temper control		
Memory		
Anxiety		
Sleep		
Other (list)		

Reminders: ❏ Review my One Page Miracle.
❏ Take my brain healthy supplements.
❏ Focus on brain healthy food.
❏ Exercise daily.

3 Things I'm Grateful for Today

1. _____

2. _____

3. _____

ANT Population *(Circle: Low/Moderate/High)*
Write down any negative thoughts and correct:

_____

Write down any challenges:

_____

DAY 7

Healing ADD Daily Journal

Time	Food and Beverages	Calories *if weight loss desired*	Healthy?	How Did I Feel After?
	Breakfast		Yes/ No	
	Snack		Yes/ No	
	Lunch		Yes/ No	
	Snack		Yes/ No	
	Dinner		Yes/ No	
	Other			

Total Calories Allowed		Total Calories Consumed	
		Total Liquid Calories Consumed	

Make it simple and find a food routine you love.

Healing ADD Daily Journal

Date:_____ Hours Slept Last Night: _____

Rate	1-10	Notes
Focus		
Organization		
Impulse control		
Worry		
Mood		
Temper control		
Memory		
Anxiety		
Sleep		
Other (list)		

Reminders:
- ❏ Review my One Page Miracle.
- ❏ Take my brain healthy supplements.
- ❏ Focus on brain healthy food.
- ❏ Exercise daily.

3 Things I'm Grateful for Today

1. _____

2. _____

3. _____

ANT Population *(Circle: Low/Moderate/High)*
Write down any negative thoughts and correct:

_____

Write down any challenges:

_____

Healing ADD Daily Journal

Time	Food and Beverages	Calories *if weight loss desired*	Healthy?	How Did I Feel After?
	Breakfast		Yes/ No	
	Snack		Yes/ No	
	Lunch		Yes/ No	
	Snack		Yes/ No	
	Dinner		Yes/ No	
	Other			

Total Calories Allowed		Total Calories Consumed	
		Total Liquid Calories Consumed	

Tip of the day: Never feel deprived by eating right. Feel deprived when you eat poorly and deprive yourself of what you want most ... your great health.

Healing ADD Daily Journal

Date:_____ Hours Slept Last Night: _____

Rate	1-10	Notes
Focus		
Organization		
Impulse control		
Worry		
Mood		
Temper control		
Memory		
Anxiety		
Sleep		
Other (list)		

Reminders: ❏ Review my One Page Miracle.
❏ Take my brain healthy supplements.
❏ Focus on brain healthy food.
❏ Exercise daily.

3 Things I'm Grateful for Today

1. _____

2. _____

3. _____

ANT Population *(Circle: Low/Moderate/High)*
Write down any negative thoughts and correct:

_____

Write down any challenges:

_____

Healing ADD Daily Journal

Time	Food and Beverages	Calories *if weight loss desired*	Healthy?	How Did I Feel After?
	Breakfast		Yes/ No	
	Snack		Yes/ No	
	Lunch		Yes/ No	
	Snack		Yes/ No	
	Dinner		Yes/ No	
	Other			

Total Calories Allowed		Total Calories Consumed	
		Total Liquid Calories Consumed	

Tip of the day: Supplement your success by knowing your type.

Healing ADD Daily Journal

DAY 10

Date:_____ **Hours Slept Last Night:** _____

Rate	1-10	Notes
Focus		
Organization		
Impulse control		
Worry		
Mood		
Temper control		
Memory		
Anxiety		
Sleep		
Other (list)		

Reminders:　❏ Review my One Page Miracle.
　　　　　　　❏ Take my brain healthy supplements.
　　　　　　　❏ Focus on brain healthy food.
　　　　　　　❏ Exercise daily.

3 Things I'm Grateful for Today

1. _____

2. _____

3. _____

ANT Population *(Circle: Low/Moderate/High)*
Write down any negative thoughts and correct:

_____

Write down any challenges:

_____

Healing ADD Daily Journal

Time	Food and Beverages	Calories *if weight loss desired*	Healthy?	How Did I Feel After?
	Breakfast		Yes/ No	
	Snack		Yes/ No	
	Lunch		Yes/ No	
	Snack		Yes/ No	
	Dinner		Yes/ No	
	Other			

Total Calories Allowed		Total Calories Consumed	
		Total Liquid Calories Consumed	

Tip of the day: People get maximally better in the 4 circles.

Healing ADD Daily Journal

DAY 11

Date:_____ Hours Slept Last Night:_____

Rate	1-10	Notes
Focus		
Organization		
Impulse control		
Worry		
Mood		
Temper control		
Memory		
Anxiety		
Sleep		
Other (list)		

Reminders: ❏ Review my One Page Miracle.
❏ Take my brain healthy supplements.
❏ Focus on brain healthy food.
❏ Exercise daily.

3 Things I'm Grateful for Today

1. _____

2. _____

3. _____

ANT Population *(Circle: Low/Moderate/High)*
Write down any negative thoughts and correct:

_____

Write down any challenges:

_____

DAY 11 Healing ADD Daily Journal

Time	Food and Beverages	Calories if weight loss desired	Healthy?	How Did I Feel After?
	Breakfast		Yes/ No	
	Snack		Yes/ No	
	Lunch		Yes/ No	
	Snack		Yes/ No	
	Dinner		Yes/ No	
	Other			

Total Calories Allowed		Total Calories Consumed	
		Total Liquid Calories Consumed	

Tip of the day: Look at your One Page Miracle every day and ask yourself if your behavior gets you what you want.

DAY 12 Healing ADD Daily Journal

Date:_____ Hours Slept Last Night: _____

Rate	1-10	Notes
Focus		
Organization		
Impulse control		
Worry		
Mood		
Temper control		
Memory		
Anxiety		
Sleep		
Other (list)		

Reminders:
- ❏ Review my One Page Miracle.
- ❏ Take my brain healthy supplements.
- ❏ Focus on brain healthy food.
- ❏ Exercise daily.

3 Things I'm Grateful for Today

1. _____

2. _____

3. _____

ANT Population *(Circle: Low/Moderate/High)*
Write down any negative thoughts and correct:

_____

Write down any challenges:

_____

Healing ADD Daily Journal

DAY 12

Time	Food and Beverages	Calories *if weight loss desired*	Healthy?	How Did I Feel After?
	Breakfast		Yes/ No	
	Snack		Yes/ No	
	Lunch		Yes/ No	
	Snack		Yes/ No	
	Dinner		Yes/ No	
	Other			

Total Calories Allowed		Total Calories Consumed	
		Total Liquid Calories Consumed	

Tip of the day: Make physical exercise
a priority for your mind.

Healing ADD Daily Journal

DAY 13

Date:_____ **Hours Slept Last Night:** _____

Rate	1-10	Notes
Focus		
Organization		
Impulse control		
Worry		
Mood		
Temper control		
Memory		
Anxiety		
Sleep		
Other (list)		

Reminders:
- ❏ Review my One Page Miracle.
- ❏ Take my brain healthy supplements.
- ❏ Focus on brain healthy food.
- ❏ Exercise daily.

3 Things I'm Grateful for Today

1. _____

2. _____

3. _____

ANT Population *(Circle: Low/Moderate/High)*
Write down any negative thoughts and correct:

_____

Write down any challenges:

_____

DAY 13 **Healing ADD Daily Journal**

Time	Food and Beverages	Calories *if weight loss desired*	Healthy?	How Did I Feel After?
	Breakfast		Yes/ No	
	Snack		Yes/ No	
	Lunch		Yes/ No	
	Snack		Yes/ No	
	Dinner		Yes/ No	
	Other			

Total Calories Allowed		Total Calories Consumed	
		Total Liquid Calories Consumed	

Tip of the day: Don't believe every stupid thought you have.

Healing ADD Daily Journal

DAY 14

Date:_____ **Hours Slept Last Night:** _____

Rate	1-10	Notes
Focus		
Organization		
Impulse control		
Worry		
Mood		
Temper control		
Memory		
Anxiety		
Sleep		
Other (list)		

Reminders:
- ❏ Review my One Page Miracle.
- ❏ Take my brain healthy supplements.
- ❏ Focus on brain healthy food.
- ❏ Exercise daily.

3 Things I'm Grateful for Today

1. _____

2. _____

3. _____

ANT Population *(Circle: Low/Moderate/High)*
Write down any negative thoughts and correct:

_____

Write down any challenges:

_____

DAY 14

Healing ADD Daily Journal

Time	Food and Beverages	Calories *if weight loss desired*	Healthy?	How Did I Feel After?
	Breakfast		Yes/ No	
	Snack		Yes/ No	
	Lunch		Yes/ No	
	Snack		Yes/ No	
	Dinner		Yes/ No	
	Other			

Total Calories Allowed		Total Calories Consumed	
		Total Liquid Calories Consumed	

Tip of the day: Use the 4 questions to save your sanity.

DAY 15 Healing ADD Daily Journal

Date:_____ Hours Slept Last Night:_____

Rate	1-10	Notes
Focus		
Organization		
Impulse control		
Worry		
Mood		
Temper control		
Memory		
Anxiety		
Sleep		
Other (list)		

Reminders:
- ❏ Review my One Page Miracle.
- ❏ Take my brain healthy supplements.
- ❏ Focus on brain healthy food.
- ❏ Exercise daily.

3 Things I'm Grateful for Today

1. _____

2. _____

3. _____

ANT Population *(Circle: Low/Moderate/High)*
Write down any negative thoughts and correct:

_____

Write down any challenges:

_____

DAY 15 **Healing ADD Daily Journal**

Time	Food and Beverages	Calories *if weight loss desired*	Healthy?	How Did I Feel After?
	Breakfast		Yes/ No	
	Snack		Yes/ No	
	Lunch		Yes/ No	
	Snack		Yes/ No	
	Dinner		Yes/ No	
	Other			

Total Calories Allowed		Total Calories Consumed	
		Total Liquid Calories Consumed	

Tip of the day: Make sleep a priority.

Healing ADD Daily Journal

DAY 16

Date:_____ Hours Slept Last Night: _____

Rate	1-10	Notes
Focus		
Organization		
Impulse control		
Worry		
Mood		
Temper control		
Memory		
Anxiety		
Sleep		
Other (list)		

Reminders: ❑ Review my One Page Miracle.
❑ Take my brain healthy supplements.
❑ Focus on brain healthy food.
❑ Exercise daily.

3 Things I'm Grateful for Today

1. _____

2. _____

3. _____

ANT Population *(Circle: Low/Moderate/High)*
Write down any negative thoughts and correct:

_____

Write down any challenges:

_____

Healing ADD Daily Journal

DAY 16

Time	Food and Beverages	Calories *if weight loss desired*	Healthy?	How Did I Feel After?
	Breakfast		Yes/ No	
	Snack		Yes/ No	
	Lunch		Yes/ No	
	Snack		Yes/ No	
	Dinner		Yes/ No	
	Other			

Total Calories Allowed		Total Calories Consumed	
		Total Liquid Calories Consumed	

Tip of the day: Balance your blood sugar to boost decision making ability.

Healing ADD Daily Journal

DAY 17

Date:_____ Hours Slept Last Night: _____

Rate	1-10	Notes
Focus		
Organization		
Impulse control		
Worry		
Mood		
Temper control		
Memory		
Anxiety		
Sleep		
Other (list)		

Reminders:
- ❑ Review my One Page Miracle.
- ❑ Take my brain healthy supplements.
- ❑ Focus on brain healthy food.
- ❑ Exercise daily.

3 Things I'm Grateful for Today

1. _____

2. _____

3. _____

ANT Population *(Circle: Low/Moderate/High)*
Write down any negative thoughts and correct:

_____

Write down any challenges:

_____

Healing ADD Daily Journal

Time	Food and Beverages	Calories *if weight loss desired*	Healthy?	How Did I Feel After?
	Breakfast		Yes/ No	
	Snack		Yes/ No	
	Lunch		Yes/ No	
	Snack		Yes/ No	
	Dinner		Yes/ No	
	Other			

Total Calories Allowed		Total Calories Consumed	
		Total Liquid Calories Consumed	

Tip of the day: Write down 3 things you are grateful for every day.

Healing ADD Daily Journal

Date:_____ Hours Slept Last Night: _____

Rate	1-10	Notes
Focus		
Organization		
Impulse control		
Worry		
Mood		
Temper control		
Memory		
Anxiety		
Sleep		
Other (list)		

Reminders: ❏ Review my One Page Miracle.
  ❏ Take my brain healthy supplements.
  ❏ Focus on brain healthy food.
  ❏ Exercise daily.

3 Things I'm Grateful for Today

1. _____

2. _____

3. _____

ANT Population *(Circle: Low/Moderate/High)*
Write down any negative thoughts and correct:

_____

Write down any challenges:

_____

Healing ADD Daily Journal

Time	Food and Beverages	Calories *if weight loss desired*	Healthy?	How Did I Feel After?
	Breakfast		Yes/ No	
	Snack		Yes/ No	
	Lunch		Yes/ No	
	Snack		Yes/ No	
	Dinner		Yes/ No	
	Other			

Total Calories Allowed		Total Calories Consumed	
		Total Liquid Calories Consumed	

Tip of the day: If you learn from your mistakes, you will make many fewer of them.

DAY 19 Healing ADD Daily Journal

Date: _____ Hours Slept Last Night: _____

Rate	1-10	Notes
Focus		
Organization		
Impulse control		
Worry		
Mood		
Temper control		
Memory		
Anxiety		
Sleep		
Other (list)		

Reminders:
- ❏ Review my One Page Miracle.
- ❏ Take my brain healthy supplements.
- ❏ Focus on brain healthy food.
- ❏ Exercise daily.

3 Things I'm Grateful for Today

1. _____

2. _____

3. _____

ANT Population *(Circle: Low/Moderate/High)*
Write down any negative thoughts and correct:

_____

Write down any challenges:

_____

Healing ADD Daily Journal

Time	Food and Beverages	Calories *if weight loss desired*	Healthy?	How Did I Feel After?
	Breakfast		Yes/ No	
	Snack		Yes/ No	
	Lunch		Yes/ No	
	Snack		Yes/ No	
	Dinner		Yes/ No	
	Other			

Total Calories Allowed		Total Calories Consumed	
		Total Liquid Calories Consumed	

Tip of the day: Simple meditations can boost your brain.

DAY 20 | Healing ADD Daily Journal

Date:_____ Hours Slept Last Night: _____

Rate	1-10	Notes
Focus		
Organization		
Impulse control		
Worry		
Mood		
Temper control		
Memory		
Anxiety		
Sleep		
Other (list)		

Reminders:
- ❑ Review my One Page Miracle.
- ❑ Take my brain healthy supplements.
- ❑ Focus on brain healthy food.
- ❑ Exercise daily.

3 Things I'm Grateful for Today

1. _____

2. _____

3. _____

ANT Population *(Circle: Low/Moderate/High)*
Write down any negative thoughts and correct:

_____

Write down any challenges:

_____

Healing ADD Daily Journal

DAY 20

Time	Food and Beverages	Calories *if weight loss desired*	Healthy?	How Did I Feel After?
	Breakfast		Yes/ No	
	Snack		Yes/ No	
	Lunch		Yes/ No	
	Snack		Yes/ No	
	Dinner		Yes/ No	
	Other			

Total Calories Allowed		Total Calories Consumed	
		Total Liquid Calories Consumed	

Tip of the day: Breathe with your belly to maintain focus and control.

Healing ADD Daily Journal

DAY 21

Date:_____ Hours Slept Last Night:_____

Rate	1-10	Notes
Focus		
Organization		
Impulse control		
Worry		
Mood		
Temper control		
Memory		
Anxiety		
Sleep		
Other (list)		

Reminders: ❏ Review my One Page Miracle.
❏ Take my brain healthy supplements.
❏ Focus on brain healthy food.
❏ Exercise daily.

3 Things I'm Grateful for Today

1. _____

2. _____

3. _____

ANT Population *(Circle: Low/Moderate/High)*

Write down any negative thoughts and correct:

_____

Write down any challenges:

_____

DAY 21

Healing ADD Daily Journal

Time	Food and Beverages	Calories *if weight loss desired*	Healthy?	How Did I Feel After?
	Breakfast		Yes/ No	
	Snack		Yes/ No	
	Lunch		Yes/ No	
	Snack		Yes/ No	
	Dinner		Yes/ No	
	Other			

Total Calories Allowed		Total Calories Consumed	
		Total Liquid Calories Consumed	

Tip of the day: Make goals for yourself as a parent.

Healing ADD Daily Journal

Date:_____ Hours Slept Last Night: _____

Rate	1-10	Notes
Focus		
Organization		
Impulse control		
Worry		
Mood		
Temper control		
Memory		
Anxiety		
Sleep		
Other (list)		

Reminders: ❏ Review my One Page Miracle.

❏ Take my brain healthy supplements.

❏ Focus on brain healthy food.

❏ Exercise daily.

3 Things I'm Grateful for Today

1. _____

2. _____

3. _____

ANT Population *(Circle: Low/Moderate/High)*
Write down any negative thoughts and correct:

_____

Write down any challenges:

_____

Healing ADD Daily Journal

Time	Food and Beverages	Calories *if weight loss desired*	Healthy?	How Did I Feel After?
	Breakfast		Yes/ No	
	Snack		Yes/ No	
	Lunch		Yes/ No	
	Snack		Yes/ No	
	Dinner		Yes/ No	
	Other			

Total Calories Allowed		Total Calories Consumed	
		Total Liquid Calories Consumed	

Tip of the day: Work on strengthening your bonds with those you love.

Healing ADD Daily Journal

Date: _____ Hours Slept Last Night: _____

Rate	1-10	Notes
Focus		
Organization		
Impulse control		
Worry		
Mood		
Temper control		
Memory		
Anxiety		
Sleep		
Other (list)		

Reminders: ❏ Review my One Page Miracle.
❏ Take my brain healthy supplements.
❏ Focus on brain healthy food.
❏ Exercise daily.

3 Things I'm Grateful for Today

1. _____

2. _____

3. _____

ANT Population *(Circle: Low/Moderate/High)*
Write down any negative thoughts and correct:

_____

Write down any challenges:

_____

Healing ADD Daily Journal

Time	Food and Beverages	Calories *if weight loss desired*	Healthy?	How Did I Feel After?
	Breakfast		Yes/ No	
	Snack		Yes/ No	
	Lunch		Yes/ No	
	Snack		Yes/ No	
	Dinner		Yes/ No	
	Other			

Total Calories Allowed		Total Calories Consumed	
		Total Liquid Calories Consumed	

Tip of the day: Children do best with clear expectations. Rules are helpful to the developing brain.

DAY 24 Healing ADD Daily Journal

Date:_____ Hours Slept Last Night: _____

Rate	1-10	Notes
Focus		
Organization		
Impulse control		
Worry		
Mood		
Temper control		
Memory		
Anxiety		
Sleep		
Other (list)		

Reminders: ❏ Review my One Page Miracle.
❏ Take my brain healthy supplements.
❏ Focus on brain healthy food.
❏ Exercise daily.

3 Things I'm Grateful for Today

1. _____

2. _____

3. _____

ANT Population *(Circle: Low/Moderate/High)*
Write down any negative thoughts and correct:

_____

Write down any challenges:

_____

DAY 24 **Healing ADD Daily Journal**

Time	Food and Beverages	Calories *if weight loss desired*	Healthy?	How Did I Feel After?
	Breakfast		Yes/ No	
	Snack		Yes/ No	
	Lunch		Yes/ No	
	Snack		Yes/ No	
	Dinner		Yes/ No	
	Other			

Total Calories Allowed		Total Calories Consumed	
		Total Liquid Calories Consumed	

*Tip of the day: Notice what you like
more than what you don't.*

Healing ADD Daily Journal

Date:_____ Hours Slept Last Night: _____

Rate	1-10	Notes
Focus		
Organization		
Impulse control		
Worry		
Mood		
Temper control		
Memory		
Anxiety		
Sleep		
Other (list)		

Reminders:
- ❏ Review my One Page Miracle.
- ❏ Take my brain healthy supplements.
- ❏ Focus on brain healthy food.
- ❏ Exercise daily.

3 Things I'm Grateful for Today

1. _____

2. _____

3. _____

ANT Population *(Circle: Low/Moderate/High)*
Write down any negative thoughts and correct:

_____

Write down any challenges:

_____

DAY 25 **Healing ADD Daily Journal**

Time	Food and Beverages	Calories *if weight loss desired*	Healthy?	How Did I Feel After?
	Breakfast		Yes/ No	
	Snack		Yes/ No	
	Lunch		Yes/ No	
	Snack		Yes/ No	
	Dinner		Yes/ No	
	Other			

Total Calories Allowed		Total Calories Consumed	
		Total Liquid Calories Consumed	

Tip of the day: Discipline in love is loving.

DAY 26 **Healing ADD Daily Journal**

Date:_____ **Hours Slept Last Night:** _____

Rate	1-10	Notes
Focus		
Organization		
Impulse control		
Worry		
Mood		
Temper control		
Memory		
Anxiety		
Sleep		
Other (list)		

Reminders: ❏ Review my One Page Miracle.
❏ Take my brain healthy supplements.
❏ Focus on brain healthy food.
❏ Exercise daily.

3 Things I'm Grateful for Today

1. _____

2. _____

3. _____

ANT Population *(Circle: Low/Moderate/High)*
Write down any negative thoughts and correct:

_____

Write down any challenges:

_____

Healing ADD Daily Journal

Time	Food and Beverages	Calories *if weight loss desired*	Healthy?	How Did I Feel After?
	Breakfast		Yes/ No	
	Snack		Yes/ No	
	Lunch		Yes/ No	
	Snack		Yes/ No	
	Dinner		Yes/ No	
	Other			

Total Calories Allowed		Total Calories Consumed	
		Total Liquid Calories Consumed	

Tip of the day: Never fight when your treatment has worn off.

DAY 27 **Healing ADD Daily Journal**

Date:_____ **Hours Slept Last Night:** _____

Rate	1-10	Notes
Focus		
Organization		
Impulse control		
Worry		
Mood		
Temper control		
Memory		
Anxiety		
Sleep		
Other (list)		

Reminders: ❑ Review my One Page Miracle.
❑ Take my brain healthy supplements.
❑ Focus on brain healthy food.
❑ Exercise daily.

3 Things I'm Grateful for Today

1. _____

2. _____

3. _____

ANT Population *(Circle: Low/Moderate/High)*
Write down any negative thoughts and correct:

_____

Write down any challenges:

_____

DAY 27

Healing ADD Daily Journal

Time	Food and Beverages	Calories *if weight loss desired*	Healthy?	How Did I Feel After?
	Breakfast		Yes/ No	
	Snack		Yes/ No	
	Lunch		Yes/ No	
	Snack		Yes/ No	
	Dinner		Yes/ No	
	Other			

Total Calories Allowed		Total Calories Consumed	
		Total Liquid Calories Consumed	

Tip of the day: Never argue with someone who is stuck.

DAY 28 **Healing ADD Daily Journal**

Date:_____ **Hours Slept Last Night:** _____

Rate	1-10	Notes
Focus		
Organization		
Impulse control		
Worry		
Mood		
Temper control		
Memory		
Anxiety		
Sleep		
Other (list)		

Reminders: ❏ Review my One Page Miracle.

❏ Take my brain healthy supplements.

❏ Focus on brain healthy food.

❏ Exercise daily.

3 Things I'm Grateful for Today

1. _____

2. _____

3. _____

ANT Population *(Circle: Low/Moderate/High)*
Write down any negative thoughts and correct:

_____

Write down any challenges:

_____

Healing ADD Daily Journal

DAY 28

Time	Food and Beverages	Calories *if weight loss desired*	Healthy?	How Did I Feel After?
	Breakfast		Yes/ No	
	Snack		Yes/ No	
	Lunch		Yes/ No	
	Snack		Yes/ No	
	Dinner		Yes/ No	
	Other			

Total Calories Allowed		Total Calories Consumed	
		Total Liquid Calories Consumed	

Tip of the day: Persist in getting help.

DAY 29   Healing ADD Daily Journal

Date:_____ Hours Slept Last Night: _____

Rate	1-10	Notes
Focus		
Organization		
Impulse control		
Worry		
Mood		
Temper control		
Memory		
Anxiety		
Sleep		
Other (list)		

Reminders: ❏ Review my One Page Miracle.
❏ Take my brain healthy supplements.
❏ Focus on brain healthy food.
❏ Exercise daily.

3 Things I'm Grateful for Today

1. _____

2. _____

3. _____

ANT Population *(Circle: Low/Moderate/High)*
Write down any negative thoughts and correct:

_____

Write down any challenges:

_____

Healing ADD Daily Journal

Time	Food and Beverages	Calories *if weight loss desired*	Healthy?	How Did I Feel After?
	Breakfast		Yes/ No	
	Snack		Yes/ No	
	Lunch		Yes/ No	
	Snack		Yes/ No	
	Dinner		Yes/ No	
	Other			

Total Calories Allowed		Total Calories Consumed	
		Total Liquid Calories Consumed	

Tip of the day: It is the smart person who seeks the best help when they have need.

DAY 30

Healing ADD Daily Journal

Date:_____ Hours Slept Last Night: _____

Rate	1-10	Notes
Focus		
Organization		
Impulse control		
Worry		
Mood		
Temper control		
Memory		
Anxiety		
Sleep		
Other (list)		

Reminders:
- ❏ Review my One Page Miracle.
- ❏ Take my brain healthy supplements.
- ❏ Focus on brain healthy food.
- ❏ Exercise daily.

3 Things I'm Grateful for Today

1. _____

2. _____

3. _____

ANT Population *(Circle: Low/Moderate/High)*
Write down any negative thoughts and correct:

_____

Write down any challenges:

_____

Healing ADD Daily Journal

Time	Food and Beverages	Calories *if weight loss desired*	Healthy?	How Did I Feel After?
	Breakfast		Yes/ No	
	Snack		Yes/ No	
	Lunch		Yes/ No	
	Snack		Yes/ No	
	Dinner		Yes/ No	
	Other			

Total Calories Allowed		Total Calories Consumed	
		Total Liquid Calories Consumed	

Tip of the day: ADD is real and when left untreated it can devastate a person's life.

Bonus Materials

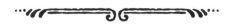

62 Best Brain Foods

1. Acai berries
2. Almonds, raw
3. Almond milk, unsweetened
4. Apples
5. Asparagus
6. Avocados
7. Bananas
8. Beans
9. Bell peppers
10. Beets
11. Blackberries
12. Blueberries
13. Bok choy
14. Brazil nuts
15. Broccoli
16. Brussels sprouts
17. Cabbage
18. Cacao, raw
19. Cauliflower
20. Chia seeds
21. Cherries
22. Chick peas
23. Chicken, skinless
24. Coconut
25. Coconut oil
26. Egg whites, DHA enriched
27. Garlic
28. Goji berries
29. Grapefruit
30. Herring
31. Grapeseed Oil
32. Kale
33. Kiwi
34. Lamb
35. Lemons
36. Lentils
37. Limes
38. Maca root
39. Olive oil
40. Onions
41. Oranges
42. Peaches
43. Pears
44. Peas
45. Plums
46. Pomegranates
47. Pumpkin seeds
48. Quinoa
49. Raspberries
50. Red grapes
51. Salmon, wild
52. Sardines
53. Sesame seeds
54. Spinach
55. Strawberries
56. Tea, green
57. Tomatoes
58. Tuna
59. Turkey, skinless
60. Walnuts
61. Water
62. Yams/sweet potatoes

Brain Healthy Shopping List

Buy organic, locally grown, unprocessed foods whenever possible. For meats, try to only buy grass fed, hormone free, and antibiotic free products.

Produce

- Acorn squash
- Apples*
- Apricots
- Artichokes
- Asparagus*
- Avocados*
- Bananas*
- Bell peppers
  (yellow, green, red, orange)*
- Beets*
- Blackberries*
- Blueberries*
- Bok choy*
- Broccoli*
- Brussels sprouts*
- Butternut squash
- Cabbage
- Cantaloupe
- Carrots
- Cauliflower
- Celery
- Cherries*
- Collard greens
- Cranberries
- Cucumbers
- Eggplant
- Grapefruit*
- Green beans
- Honeydew
- Jicama
- Kale
- Kiwi*
- Leeks
- Lemons*
- Lettuce
- Limes*
- Mangoes
- Mesclun
- Mushrooms
- Mustard greens
- Nectarines
- Okra
- Olives
- Onions
- Oranges*
- Papaya
- Parsnips
- Peaches*
- Pears*
- Peas*
- Plums
- Pomegranates*
- Pumpkin
- Radish
- Raspberries*
- Plums*
- Red grapes*
- Snap peas
- Soy beans*
- Spaghetti squash
- Spinach*
- Strawberries*
- Swiss chard
- Tangerines
- Tomatoes*
- Turnips
- Watercress
- Yams/sweet potatoes*
- Zucchini

Meats & Seafood

- Anchovies
- Beef, lean cuts
- Chicken, skinless*
- Chicken, ground white meat
- Clams
- Crab
- Flounder
- Haddock
- Halibut
- Herring*
- Lamb
- Lobster
- Mackerel
- Oysters
- Salmon, wild*
- Sardines
- Scallops
- Sea bass
- Shrimp
- Snapper
- Swordfish
- Trout
- Tuna*
- Turkey, skinless*
- Turkey, ground white meat

Beverages

- ❏ Almond milk, unsweetened*
- ❏ Coconut water
- ❏ Coffee (decaf)
- ❏ Rice milk, unsweetened
- ❏ Tea, black (decaf)
- ❏ Tea, green* (decaf)
- ❏ Tea, herbal (decaf)
- ❏ Water*

Beans

- ❏ Black beans*
- ❏ Black-eyed peas
- ❏ Fava beans
- ❏ Kidney beans
- ❏ Pinto beans*
- ❏ Garbanzo beans*
- ❏ Lentils*
- ❏ Lima beans
- ❏ Navy beans
- ❏ Organic soybeans (edamame)
- ❏ Split peas
- ❏ White beans

Nuts, Seeds & Oils

- ❏ Almonds, raw*
- ❏ Coconut oil
- ❏ Cashews
- ❏ Flaxseed oil
- ❏ Hazelnuts
- ❏ Olive oil*
- ❏ Olive oil spray
- ❏ Almond butter
- ❏ Almonds
- ❏ Pecans
- ❏ Pistachios
- ❏ Pumpkin seeds
- ❏ Quinoa
- ❏ Sesame seeds
- ❏ Sunflower seeds
- ❏ Walnuts*

Spices, Seasonings & Dressings

- ❏ Balsamic vinegar
- ❏ Basil
- ❏ Cinnamon
- ❏ Curry/turmeric
- ❏ Garlic
- ❏ Ginger
- ❏ Marinara sauce, low-sugar
- ❏ Marjoram
- ❏ Mustard
- ❏ Oregano
- ❏ Rosemary
- ❏ Saffron
- ❏ Sage
- ❏ Thyme

Snacks & Health Foods

- ❏ Dark chocolate, low sugar
- ❏ Dried veggies, no added oil
- ❏ Stevia
- ❏ Xylitol

Frozen Foods

- ❏ Fruits
- ❏ Chicken breasts
- ❏ Seafood
- ❏ Turkey burgers
- ❏ Salmon burgers
- ❏ Veggies

Refrigerated Products

- ❏ Eggs, DHA-rich
- ❏ Guacamole
- ❏ Hummus
- ❏ Salsa
- ❏ Organic Tofu

* Note: these foods should be used sparingly.

Eco-Friendly Brain Healthy Eating Tips

Not all foods are created equal, not even brain healthy foods. Part of brain healthy eating is being smart about choosing the foods that are the best not only for our brains and bodies but also for the environment. When shopping for the brain healthy fish included on the Brain Healthy Shopping List, choose the most eco-friendly. The following recommendations come from the *Monterey Bay Aquarium Seafood Watch* program. You can download pocket guides to more types of fish at:

http://www.seafoodwatch.org/cr/cr_seafoodwatch/download.aspx

BRAIN HEALTHY FISH	EAT THESE OFTEN	OK TO EAT SOMETIMES	DON'T EAT THESE
Clams	Farmed	Wild	
Crab	Dungeness, Stone	Blue, King (U.S.), Snow	
Flounder		Pacific	Atlantic
Halibut	Pacific		Atlantic
Herring		Atlantic	
Lobster	Spiny (U.S.)	American/Maine	Spiny (Brazil)
Oysters	Farmed	Wild	
Salmon	Wild (Alaska)	Wild (Washington)	Wild (California, Oregon) Farmed, including Atlantic
Scallops	Farmed Off-bottom	Sea	
Seabass			Chilean seabass
Shrimp	Pink (Oregon)	U.S. or Canada	Imported
Snapper			Red
Swordfish		U.S.	Imported
Trout	Rainbow (farmed)		
Tuna	Albacore including canned white tuna (pole/troll, U.S. and British Columbia); Skipjack including canned light tuna (pole/troll)	Bigeye, Yelllowfin (pole/troll); canned white/Albacore (pole troll except U.S. and British Columbia)	Albacore, Bigeye, Yellowfin (longline); Bluefin, Tongol; canned (except pole/troll)

Additional Resources

Amen Clinics Supplement Club

Enroll in the Amen Clinics Supplement Club
http://store.amenclinics.com

BrainFit Life Online Community

http://mybrainfitlife.com

Register for this online program where you can:

- Assess your brain
- Mental workouts tailored specifically to your brain's needs
- Track your progress
- Keep an online food and brain health journal
- Find brain healthy recipes for breakfast, lunch, dinner, snacks, and even desserts
- Create a "My Motivation Page" to help keep you focused
- Create an online version of your "One-Page Miracle"
- Find interactive exercises to help you kill the ANTs
- Find proven stress-management techniques
- Find tips to bust your barriers
- Community of thousands of like-minded members to get brain healthy together

Healing ADD through Food

A cookbook from nurse Tana Amen that shows you how to make brain healthy meals the whole family will love.